Valerie Bingham was born 
educated at Latymer Gramm
at R.A.D.A before the money

She met Jack at an amateur _____ they
married in 1959. They have tw_____ currently reside in
Ludlow, Shropshire.

Valerie has always had a passion for poetry and prose, and
has had pieces published. However, this is her first full
length book, prompted by her experiences in dealing with
her husband's illness. She found the writing process to be
cathartic, and hopes the book will help others in similar
circumstances.

THE ROCKY ROAD TO LA-LA-LAND

(A Descent into Alzheimer's)

Valerie Bingham

THE ROCKY ROAD TO LA-LA-LAND

(A Descent into Alzheimer's)

Olympia Publishers
London

www.olympiapublishers.com
OLYMPIA PAPERBACK EDITION

Copyright © Valerie Bingham 2014

The right of Valerie Bingham to be identified as author of
this work has been asserted in accordance with sections 77 and
78 of the Copyright, Designs and Patents Act 1988.

All Rights Reserved

No reproduction, copy or transmission of this publication
may be made without written permission.
No paragraph of this publication may be reproduced,
copied or transmitted save with the written permission of the
publisher, or in accordance with the provisions
of the Copyright Act 1956 (as amended).

Any person who commits any unauthorised act in relation to
this publication may be liable to criminal
prosecution and civil claims for damage.

A CIP catalogue record for this title is
available from the British Library.

ISBN: 978-1-84897-480-7

First Published in 2014

Olympia Publishers
60 Cannon Street
London
EC4N 6NP

Printed in Great Britain

This book is dedicated to all the people
who have given Jack tender loving care during his illness.

In particular, Ashfield House, Bradeney House,
and Helena Lane Day Care

Acknowledgments

My grateful thanks to Rachel and Matthew Bingham for all their support and practical help during the making of this book.

1

Dropped Stitch

I have just finished talking to my husband Jack on the phone. It wasn't a very satisfactory conversation – it seldom is these days but I can picture him secure and cosy in his residential home. Christmas 2010 came and went and now there were the interminable bank holidays to get through. This was our first Christmas apart in fifty-one years, except when I gave birth on Christmas Eve to our youngest son in hospital. It wasn't too bad actually – Christmas that is. I finally got custody of the remote control and pulled my armchair nearer the fire, toasted my toes and watched my favourite TV programmes with a box of chocolates and a bottle of ginger wine close to hand.

Mind you, it wasn't quite what I had envisaged. The plan had been to travel by train to my youngest son and his family in Hove and then to my other son in London on Boxing Day, finally meeting up with my niece on the 27th, but some awful weather had put paid to all that. I had been invited to have dinner with Jack in his home but had no means of getting there as he was in another town. More of that later.

As a turkey for one person was out of the question, I roasted a small partridge with all the trimmings and finished my meal with the remains of a three-day-old trifle. That is the kind of thing that happens when you are catering for one and can't bear to waste food.

We have been a long time getting to this point and have leapt many hurdles since I first realised there was something wrong with him, Alzheimer's, like childbirth, is a different experience for everyone. With childbirth, some have a quick, violent labour, while others go on seemingly forever, but the outcome is usually a healthy baby. Jack's illness was of the seemingly forever kind; the outcome was that an intelligent, even-tempered man had taken seventeen years to turn into a stranger living in a world of his own. But it hasn't been all doom and gloom and we have had some good times on the way.

We originally came from Enfield in Middlesex, or north London as we are supposed to call it these days. In 1965 we moved to Hove in Sussex but in 1989, when Jack was 57, the car insurance firm he worked for was taken over and he was made redundant, or as good as – he was offered a transfer to Southampton but that didn't hold any appeal for us.

When the children were young, we used to go on long holidays, which is how we discovered the delightful market town of Ludlow in Shropshire. We always said we would like to retire there one day. Now it looked as if that day had come, earlier than we expected but what the hell – we put our house on the market. The timing wasn't great, it was the beginning of a recession and house prices were dropping overnight. Brighton and Hove became bed-sit land, shops and hotels were closing and the lawns of the beautiful Brighton Pavilion became a mecca for alcoholics. The beaches were strewn with needles as the drug problem escalated. We couldn't wait to move out, but wait we had to – for two-and-a-half years.

Hardly anyone viewed our property and we were thankful when a young couple offered us a price that we would have turned down as ludicrous at the outset. We accepted immediately, but the weeks before we exchanged contracts were agony. Our buyers both worked for Sussex University, which was shedding staff; it only needed one of them to lose their job for our sale to go belly-up. Fortunately for them and us this didn't transpire, and we moved to Ludlow at Easter 1992.

The removal van broke down on the motorway (the first time ever, they said). We were getting ringing tones in the kitchen but as our phone was on the van we couldn't answer them. We had no idea what was going on or where all our worldly goods were. We sat on the floor of the front room eating fish and chips while our cat, who appeared to be suffering a nervous breakdown, ignored the fish and prowled the house emitting blood-curdling yowls before getting himself shut in a cupboard. The van eventually arrived at 6pm and the men worked their socks off getting in our furniture. We left the cat in the cupboard. It seemed kinder somehow, but it didn't make for a very auspicious start!

After about eighteen months we joined the local amateur dramatic society. Jack and I have always been interested in the theatre and it has been a strong bond between us over the years. In fact we first met at a theatrical society in Enfield. Although I hadn't immediately been bowled over by his looks and personality, I was impressed with his acting ability (people join a theatre company for many reasons, not necessarily because they have talent-rather like The X-Factor). I always said to Jack that if he hadn't been able to act, our relationship would never have got off the ground.

The Ludlow society was always short of men, so it wasn't long before Jack was cast in a play. He possessed a near-photographic memory, which is ironic seeing the way things have turned out. He only had to read a script a few times to be almost word perfect. I envied him this gift, because I had to study hard to learn my lines.

As was our usual custom I offered to hear his lines – and was surprised at how often he stumbled or improvised, which was quite out of character. Even when the show went on I felt uneasy for him; he appeared to be struggling, although he didn't take a prompt in the three performances. When I tactfully alluded to this he hotly denied he had a problem and said he was concentrating on his Welsh accent.

Looking back, I think this was the first indication that something wasn't right. Was this the crucial period when his brain dropped a stitch and slowly, very slowly, his head started to unravel?

2

Holidays and Hobbies

Moving house is traumatic at the best of times let alone moving halfway across the country. It took us a while to feel really settled and make new friends but I finally thought we were getting there. I was more than happy pottering about in our lovely new garden, far bigger than our previous one, but I sensed Jack was rather at a loose end. Apart from the aforementioned theatre company he didn't know how to fill his time. He was used to playing sports; in the early days, football and cricket and latterly golf; but there was a waiting list for the local golf club. It was some while before he found a sponsor and finally became a member. At last he was able to play as often as he pleased and take part in occasional away matches.

Between redundancy and the two-and-a-half years it took to sell our house he had endeavoured to find work- if only part-time. Worthing golf club took him on for one day a week in their pro shop; he was only paid a pittance and it wasn't long before they replaced him with a student who was willing to work for even less money. The Job Centre wasn't much help, saying their books were full of people like him – middle aged and middle management. Now, here in Shropshire, he was almost sixty-two and he must have felt on the scrap heap.

Our original intention had been to open a shop but the meagre profit we made on our house put paid to that idea, so instead we took a stall at the antiques and flea market. It only took place on Sundays and we were more flea than antiques: we sold books, prints and odd pieces of china. Jack took care of the book side of things and I hunted out china at car-boot sales and charity shops. Those were the days when people weren't so aware of the true value of their possessions and there were real bargains to be had. I can't say it was a living, more of a hobby, but it was very interesting- although not much fun in the winter months as it was in the open air.

We decided the time had come to take a holiday, so we booked with a company that did tours in the Scottish Highlands. Their head office was in Glasgow but they had a sub-office in Hereford and had hotels at all the well-known lochs. As they practically took you from door to door it required little effort on our part. Our hotel was at Loch Lomond and we thoroughly enjoyed the stay, so a year or so later we booked for another one in a different location – but things didn't go so smoothly this time.

The coach took us on daily sightseeing trips and dropped us off at various places with strict instructions to be back at a certain time and place. I don't like wearing a watch so I used to leave that side of things to Jack, but I soon realised I had better pay attention as he often forgot the time, and in some instances the pick-up point. We would end up frantically looking for one of our fellow passengers in order to check when we were due back.

On one occasion we had a whole day in Edinburgh and went to a place on Princes Street for coffee. The restaurant was on the third floor and boasted magnificent views of the city. It was pretty crowded so I secured a table while Jack queued up for refreshments, but when he came back he had forgotten his sugar and had cheese scones and jam I laughed about it and offered to exchange the scones but he got all huffy and proceeded to spread jam on his cheese scone, as if to defy me. To change the subject I pointed out the large notice forbidding people to go on the balconies because they were unsafe. Shortly afterwards I nipped to the ladies, but when I returned there was no sign of him. To my horror he was out on the balcony, happily taking photos.

Another time, in Fort William, he announced he had lost his wallet. We revisited all the shops we had been to but nobody could help us. In the end we went to the police station and left our names, telephone number and address, in the hope that someone would hand it in. Jack seemed curiously unconcerned about this, but I was worried that I didn't have enough money to cover the rest of the holiday and had great difficulty ascertaining what credit cards had been in the wallet. I was very relieved to find it on the floor of the coach when we returned; it must have fallen from his coat when he took it down from the luggage rack.

Meal times presented problems too, as he instantly forgot what he had ordered from the menu and related stories that he had previously regaled our dining companions with the evening before. When I tried to jokingly deflect him from this, he flew at me. I don't know who was the more embarrassed, our friends or me.

One evening we went for a stroll around the hotel garden, but as it grew colder I suggested we go back inside for a drink. Jack insisted we go through the back entrance, which we had never done before. After practically forcing the door open we were met with a loud alarm and a posse of staff. It took some explaining and I couldn't look them in the eye next morning at breakfast.

All these things sound so trivial but I knew in my heart it was not his normal behaviour. But when we returned home he was more like his old self and I began to think I was making a mountain out of a molehill. Did he sense I was watching him? Was I making him nervous?

One of the things I have learnt over the years is that you start to think that everything is your fault. If he couldn't find something, I must have moved it. If he went down the road for a newspaper, milk or to post a letter, and forgot, then I hadn't explained things properly. His excuses were so plausible that I really believed him.

I was finally convinced that it wasn't my imagination when I was asked to direct a Neil Simon play called Barefoot in the Park. I cast Jack as the telephone man. It was a small part, right up his street, and I fully expected him to steal the scene. Briefly the plot is about a young pair of newlyweds who buy their first flat in New York. The flat is up umpteen flights of stairs and the elevator doesn't work, and the running joke is that all their visitors arrive in a state of collapse. The play opens on a bare stage with the woman attempting to decorate as the telephone man arrives to install the phone. Jack captured the Bronx accent beautifully and did some inspired business about being exhausted, but he kept forgetting his lines.

Rehearsals became chaotic because not only were his lines all over the place but he couldn't remember his moves, in spite of marking them in his script. I went over the same ground with him again and again but it was of no use because by the time the next rehearsal came around, we were back to square one.

Between the first and second scenes the flat had to be transformed with the addition of a small kitchen, furniture, curtains, pictures and plants. It was not an easy task and would have been better had it happened in the longer time between acts, but playwrights never think of things like that. Our theatre had no curtains, so rather than have the stage hands floundering around in semi-darkness I decide to make a feature of the scene change. I had them all dressed in sweatshirts printed with the logo of Bloomingdale's, the famous New York store, and played 'busy' music accompanied by a purple lighting effect. The intention was that there was always something for the audience to watch. It should have worked perfectly.

At the technical rehearsal – a run-through to test the staging – we tried the change several times but something always went wrong. I couldn't understand why, until the stage manager took me aside and, with barely suppressed irritation, explained it was all Jack's fault: he hadn't a clue as to what he was supposed to be doing. Happily on the night everyone covered for him, and the audience gave their hard work a round of applause.

I knew then that he wasn't to be trusted with anything complicated. It grieved me terribly because he was such a good actor with a wonderful feel for comedy – I didn't want to think that this might be his swansong.

After that we coasted along as before but I couldn't help wondering what was coming next. As it happened, I didn't have long to wait. Our youngest son, Miles, and his partner

Michelle had moved from Hove to a village in the West Sussex countryside. They were eager for us to see their new home so Jack drove us there for a short break in the summer. Miles took us on a tour of the area at the weekend but the couple had to be back at work on Monday, so we were left to our own devices for three days.

We intended to have a day in Brighton and were ready for an early start, when Jack said he would just pop out for a paper and petrol There was a little row of shops and a garage quite near so I assumed he was going there, but he didn't come back. I waited for ages and stood outside the front door looking for him; we didn't have mobile phones then.

I pictured him driving around in circles and getting further and further away. Should I call the police? Jack would be furious if he turned up five minutes later. I didn't like to ring Miles at work and anyway, what could he do? Finally I stuck a note on the front door in case Jack came back and went to a triangle of grass with an A-road and a couple of B-roads running round it. Fortunately there was a bench, so I sat there trying to look in three directions at once in the hope that Jack would drive past, although how I was going to attract his attention I had no idea. After an hour I gave up.

By now I was sick with worry and convinced that Jack was completely lost. My only hope was that we were near a large windmill. Surely that would stick in his mind? He could ask someone for directions to it – but then again Jack was a man and hated asking for help.

Eventually I heard a car draw up. I rushed to the door. I was very good – I didn't scream, "Where have you been?" much as I wanted to. He looked tired and strained so I told him to sit in the garden and I'd bring him out a cup of tea. We sipped our tea and I waited for an explanation, no matter how bizarre, but he never said a word. Perhaps he didn't realise he had been gone for two-and-a-half hours!

3

Seasonal Celebrations

If there's one thing I've learnt over the years it's to not listen to your friends but to go with your gut instinct. I began expressing my misgivings to one or two close friends and they sought to comfort me. "My husband never hears what he doesn't want to hear," said one.

"I'm just as bad," said another. "I lose my shopping list, and I'm always going into a room and then forgetting what I've come in for."

The times I've heard that one! Yes, we all have our 'senior' moments, but they don't happen that often. They also told me of relatives and of friends of friends who were experiencing similar problems that would have been funny if they weren't so tragic. They told me of one fashion-conscious elderly lady who had come downstairs one day with all her make-up done with biro. Another friend said that when she took her elderly aunt out for coffee, she had stood up in the middle of the restaurant and announced at the top of her voice that she was going to the toilet. She was gone for ages and eventually her niece went to look for her, fearing she had been taken ill, "Alright, I'm coming, I'm coming," came a voice from the cubicle in ringing tones, adding in an Edith Evans voice, "I'm just wiping my arse."

Jack wasn't as bad as that, so perhaps there was still hope. But I still thought he was in need of professional help.

His skill as an actor wasn't helping matters, either; he was capable of giving an Oscar-winning performance when attempting to cover up a lapse, and almost had me believing him.

As an example, some eighteen months previously he joined the list of Women's Institute speakers. The WI is big in this part of the country; nearly every village has one, and the smaller ones amalgamate to share the cost when they have a speaker. Jack's most popular talk was on the old-time music halls and he got plenty of engagements. I was pleased he had found a new interest and it was going so well.

But now I started getting agitated phone calls from WI ladies saying he hadn't arrived and they were all sitting there waiting for him. I tried to fob them of; saying he was coming and would probably arrive any minute, but all the time I imagined him driving along unlit country lanes, getting in a panic and possibly having an accident. When he came home from one such engagement I told him of the phone call and he assured me he had arrived, if a little late, and there had been fog on the road. Another time he said they hadn't given him the correct directions. I know for a fact that in one instance he had never got to the village hall, because the chairwoman had phoned me at 8pm and again at 10. But when Jack came home, at a feasible time, he told me the talk had gone very well, and even embellished it by saying there were thirty-five members present. When I challenged him, he stomped off to bed in a huff and refused to say another word about it.

A few weeks later I was emptying the rubbish bin and spotted a crumpled letter with the WI heading on it. I smoothed it out and read that in accordance with their policy, as there had been more than two complaints made against him they were striking him off their register. My stomach lurched and I felt heartbroken for him, but also very hurt. Had that happened to me I would have rushed straight to him with the letter and poured my heart out, but Jack being Jack couldn't confide in me- his wife of more than forty years.

Shortly afterwards he suddenly announced that he wasn't doing any more talks as it was becoming a bore.

I don't know why I didn't say then that I knew the truth. I suppose it would have meant confessing that I'd read his letter. I could guess what his response would have been: "Well, if you know so much about it, why are you bothering to discuss it with me?" Once again he would turn the tables and make out it was somehow my fault.

For several years at Christmas we had been involved in putting on an entertainment for a local pub. They held a goose dinner in December and it was a lovely occasion. Ticket only, it was like a large family get-together. The evening started with a quartet of carol singers, and then the landlord would say grace and we'd all sit down to a sumptuous five-course meal. After coffee Jack and I did readings from Dickens or anything with a seasonal theme. The audience, well-oiled by now, were always very appreciative.

On the strength of this, we were engaged for a Burns Night by another pub. We met up with a chap called Andrew who was going to be the MC for the evening. The landlord was determined to make it a genuine Burns occasion with the piping in of the haggis and a pianist as further back-up. We met up in the pub for a couple of rehearsals and were given lunch and a few drinks, which was one up on play rehearsals where you were lucky to get a cup of coffee.

One of our tasks was for Jack to make a speech to 'The Ladies' and I was to reply in a similar vein on my gender's behalf. He wrote his speech and handed it to me because I had to allude to what he had written. When I read it I was dismayed to find he had wandered off the subject. It really didn't make a lot of sense. Jack was usually good at writing and had several one-act plays to his credit, which had been performed at fringe theatres in London and Brighton. The New Playwrights Network had published a full-length play, and his greatest achievement was to have had one performed on Radio 4.

I tactfully suggested he should have another go at it, but his second draft wasn't much better. I told him it wasn't suitable and he flew into a rage and said if I was so clever then I should write it myself so I did just that, trying to incorporate the odd nugget from the original and then I wrote my own speech replying to myself.

At our final rehearsal he got in a muddle and I could see that Andrew was losing patience with him. I did my best to make it simple by photocopying the script in large print, colour coding and underlining headings, and prayed it would be alright on the night. But of course it wasn't.

They were a tricky audience and, having consumed a large amount of whisky, were in a skittish mood. They loved the piper and joined in the singing but were reluctant to settle down and listen to poetry and speeches. I could see Jack getting uptight and he began shuffling his script, which got out of order. Andrew was looking daggers. I was trying to prompt him under my breath, and what should have been a great evening turned out to be a nightmare. To cap it all, Andrew asked me if Jack had been drinking beforehand. It goes without saying that we weren't invited back the following year.

To be perfectly honest I was beginning to feel ashamed of Jack. He was letting me down as well as himself. By now I thought I knew what was wrong with him but we had no diagnosis and mental illness is not always obvious to outsiders. Besides, he could be perfectly normal for weeks at a time, and Jack had always had difficulty with certain words at the best of times. These included "Sorry", "I don't understand" and "It's my fault".

Now his wretched pride was driving a wedge between us. If just once he could admit he was confused or couldn't cope I would have melted and done everything in my power to support him, but that was never going to happen. We just stumbled on from one mini-disaster to another – but looming on the horizon was a major crisis which was to affect our lives for several years.

4

Cancer

In late 2003 I learned that the founder of another local theatre company had died from cancer. The members wanted to put on a concert in his memory and I was asked to direct a one-act play by Chekov for them, called The Bear. Apparently it was a play the deceased had always wanted to produce. They thought it would be a nice gesture to include it as part of the memorial event.

As I knew most of the members I was only too happy to oblige, and so we began rehearsing. The programme consisted of scenes from some of the founder's earlier productions, interspersed with light-hearted musical items and finishing with The Bear. It wasn't long before I was asked to 'just take a look" at such and such, and could I suggest some movements for a comic song? They were also struggling with some of the scenes that had originally been performed in the round and now had to be adapted for a normal stage. Almost before I knew it I was overseeing the whole production, but that was fine by me and Jack attended some of the rehearsals.

During this time I had a routine mammogram and had thought no more about it until I received a letter asking me to come in for another one. I was rather surprised, but as I felt perfectly well and had no sign of a lump I didn't take it too seriously. Also I knew of several people who'd had recalls in the past which had turned out to be nothing.

The hospital was 30 miles away in Shrewsbury. Jack drove me but took a wrong turning, so I arrived late for my appointment and in a bit of a tizzy. I calmed down though when I saw how many people were waiting to be seen. I don't know if it was deliberate on the hospitals part, but after a second mammogram I was last to be called in to see the specialist. He put my previous mammogram up on the screen and pointed out a small white dot. Then he showed me the latest one, which now had several fine threads attached to it.

The doctor gave me a physical examination and said he could feel a small lump, and then asked me to follow him into the next room for a biopsy. I caught a brief glimpse of Jack and gave him the thumbs down sign, before being whisked away by the breast nurse. I knew it was going to be painful when she stood at my head and two nurses pinioned my arms to the table. As I tried to explain to Jack later, imagine someone inserting a large needle into your testicle. In my ancient Pears encyclopaedia it states that this procedure is normally done under anaesthetic, but I suppose these days it's considered too time-consuming.

The breast nurse led me back to Jack and told him to get me a nice cup of tea while I waited for the result. Jack returned a couple of minutes later saying he couldn't find the canteen, so the nurse took him by the arm and said she would show him where it was. I think she suspected there was something not quite right about him. Jack returned with the tea, which tasted absolutely vile because he had put in sugar and the bag was still lurking in the bottom of the mug.

I drank as much as I could stomach before we were both asked to see the specialist to discuss the result. I don't think Jack had the foggiest idea it was going to be bad news.

Sure enough, the specialist explained that the test had proved positive for cancer. I had a carcinoma in my right breast and would have to undergo a lumpectomy, but he would do his best to save my nipple. Then he told us the same information again and left the room, while the nurse went over everything for a third time. They obviously know that once you hear the word cancer your mind goes totally blank and you can't take anything else in. Jack remained impassive; he didn't realise the implications and showed no more emotion than if I'd been diagnosed with an ingrown toenail.

We got into the car. It was dark now and raining, Jack got lost at the very first roundabout. I sat there shivering, icy cold with shock, while he shouted at me for not pointing out the turn-off. I remember thinking I must be the only woman in the world to have her husband rail at her after being given a life-threatening diagnosis. I'd like to say he was suffering from shock, but things went from bad to worse when I said I couldn't cook tonight and we'd have to make do with fish and chips. At the chip shop he parked the car much too close to another and asked me if I had enough room to get out. He was about to send me out in the pouring rain to buy fish and chips – unbelievable!

The next day was the dress rehearsal for the show, which frankly was a blessing as it took my mind off what lay ahead. I was full of feverish energy and excelled myself as I dashed hither and thither without time to think. In a brief lull, one of the cast asked me how I had got on at the hospital. She was shocked when I told her the outcome. From then on the news spread like wildfire. Everyone came and hugged me and wished me well and said they would understand if 1 didn't come to the show the next evening, but I wasn't going to miss it for anything.

It was very well received and afterwards someone made a speech thanking me for all my help. They presented me with a bouquet of flowers and a huge silver balloon saying 'Thank You'. It was very touching.

This was the Saturday and I only had one day left to pack, phone my sons and make final preparations for going in on Monday. I was concerned about leaving Jack on his own, but Miles said he'd arranged a few days off and would arrive on Tuesday – the day of the op. The phone never stopped ringing that Sunday with well-wishers and people commenting about the show, and in the end I was exhausted and left Jack to handle any further calls. He was very terse with them and finally left the phone off the hook, but by then I was too weary to care.

On the way to the hospital in Telford, Jack suddenly turned off the road and we ended up trying to navigate out of an industrial estate. A man came out to speak to us and, seeing my distress, jumped in his car and led us back to the main road, for which I was very grateful. We finally got to our destination and I must admit I was relieved to kiss Jack goodbye and climb into bed, my flowers and balloon on the bedside locker. What the ward sister made of the message I have no idea – she probably thought it was a bit premature.

Everything was out of my hands now. All the angst of the past few days disappeared and I slept like a baby. True, there were several interruptions when I was weighed, re-examined and asked to fill in a form, but in between I caught up on my sleep. I couldn't have felt more content if I'd been staying at the Ritz.

Even the thought of the operation next day didn't worry me.

Tuesday morning came and at some unearthly hour I was wheeled into the bowels of the hospital for my op, but it all went well and I still had my nipple thank goodness. I woke up to find Jack and Miles at my bedside. I couldn't help noticing that most of my fellow patients had drains attached to them, but I was unencumbered. Perhaps I looked too unscathed because I soon realised that Jack was assuming that, as I would be out in a couple more days, we could go straight back to our usual routine.

The next day a nurse came and told me with a beaming smile that as I was doing so well I could leave hospital a day early. She was very surprised when I promptly burst into tears; clearly not the reaction she had been expecting, but she didn't know of my circumstances at home. I knew Jack wasn't capable of looking after me properly. The nurse asked if I wanted to see the almoner or the hospital chaplain – but I didn't want to make a fuss and settled for a cup of tea instead.

The next morning I woke feeling uncomfortable, and putting my hand on my nightie found it covered in blood. Within a minute I had been surrounded by screens. The registrar came in with a retinue of nurses and did some sort of patch-up job, warning me if it happened again I'd be back in theatre first thing the next morning.

That had put paid to me going home on time. Miles had been intending to drive me home, but as he now had to go back to work he arranged for my friend, Patricia, known as Paddy, to give me a lift later that day. (The thought of Jack picking me up and probably getting lost was not to be contemplated – my nerves wouldn't stand it.)

Paddy arrived and I said my farewells and we set off for home, every bump in the road causing me discomfort. When we got back I had to fish for my key as Jack wasn't in, but he turned up twenty minutes later with a beautiful pot plant which I assumed he'd been out to buy. But when I read the label I saw it was from my eldest son and family in London. Where Jack had been and what had induced him to go out I shall never know.

Paddy made a pot of tea as I got into bed, feebly waving a prescription for painkillers given to me by the hospital; I still laugh when I remember how she snatched it from under Jack's nose and said that she would be the one to go to the chemist. She clearly knew the score.

After she went home I realised that the hollow feeling in my stomach was not caused by her departure but by hunger. I explained to Jack that I'd only had a small bowl of cereal at 7am and it was now two and I was starving. I tried to think of something simple and asked for a cheese and tomato sandwich. After an age he appeared with a tray which held three tea plates. One contained sliced bread, the second a lump of cheese and the third held sliced tomatoes. So pulling myself upright, I proceeded to make up my own sandwich.

Jack said he hoped I'd be up tomorrow, but he was in for a disappointment as I'd been given strict instructions to stay in bed for two days. The following day, realising we were in danger of starving, I sent him off to have a meal in a cafe and bring me back a baked potato from the takeaway.

Luckily my friends rallied round with gifts of mini pizzas, tinned soup and cakes, and we muddled through until I was on my feet again. I can smile about it now but it didn't seem funny at the time.

Now I had to begin three weeks of radiotherapy, but fortunately I was able to attend via hospital transport.

This was an adventure in itself as we picked up other patients on the way, and I saw parts of the county I didn't even know existed. We went through wind, snow, frost and flooding. One morning I saw an old lady taking a large pig for a walk; another day a man was giving his ferrets an airing. I wouldn't have seen that in Brighton!

The radiotherapy was painless and the League of Friends sold the best doughnuts I have ever tasted, but the trouble was that my immune system had been temporarily destroyed. I seldom get a cold but I had several bad ones that year, plus a chest infection, and I wasn't allowed to do the garden without gloves in case I got a scratch and it became infected. Poor old Jack found himself hoovering, making beds and carrying shopping, although I still did all of the cooking. It was a difficult time made worse by an ongoing problem that just refused to clear up.

5

Impasse

When the surgeon operated on my breast he also took ten glands from under my right arm and three of them turned out to be cancerous. I tried not to think of them coursing around my body and turning up in my liver or brain, but I was put on tamoxifen, which was supposed to help counteract such a thing happening, so all I could do was to keep my fingers crossed.

Although my breast healed quickly with barely a scar, the wound under my arm refused to close. I now realised why so many patients in my ward had been put on drains, and can't for the life of me think why I hadn't had one too. As a consequence, the wound kept weeping and puffing up. I had to return to hospital at frequent intervals to have it siphoned off with a large needle, which was time-consuming and extremely painful.

I was bemoaning the fact to my GP, complaining that the journey was a nightmare with Jack's predisposition for getting lost, when he suggested I have a word at reception and get the phone number for Community Cars. I can't speak highly enough of this organisation; the drivers get very little remuneration and all you have to pay is their petrol money, which works out far cheaper than a taxi They are such nice people, mostly retired, and will take you to hospital or the doctor's surgery and wait for you no matter how long it takes, and then bring you home.

I'm sure there is something similar in most parts of the country and it's almost a necessity in rural areas, so don't hesitate to ask if you need their services. Jack used to come with me and we usually had a meal in the hospital restaurant. I would offer to treat the driver, although they generally declined. Jack so much enjoyed these 'outings' that a year or so later the driver and I watched in amazement as he got out of the front seat and crossed the road, went into our house and shut the front door – completely forgetting about me in the back of the car and the reason we had gone to the hospital in the first place.

Rather like hospital transport we had our moments, like the day we got caught in a flood and Jack had to be persuaded to stand up to his knees in water to help the driver push the car onto dry land. Another time the car broke down and the driver tried to get us a taxi, but they were all tied up doing school runs and we waited for more than an hour for a breakdown truck. I usually wore trousers on these occasions but in this instance I had on a tight skirt. I was highly embarrassed as I hitched my skirt above my knees, and Jack and the driver grabbed my bottom and heaved me up into the cab of the truck. Needless to say we didn't get to the hospital on that day.

But to get back to my ongoing problem I had to change my dressing twice a day and as it was in such an awkward position I couldn't do it myself; so Jack had to help me. I begged him to be careful with regard to hygiene, but Jack's idea of scrubbing up was to dangle his hands under tepid water and I don't think soap entered into the equation.

Whether it was his fault or not, it very soon got infected. I awoke one morning feeling as if someone had placed a golf ball under my arm overnight, and sure enough it was all swollen up and red.

The doctor saw me straight away – that was the thing about having had cancer, you only had to say the magic word and you were fast-forwarded into the surgery. He put me on antibiotics and the infection cleared up but did nothing to dry the wound. Finally the hospital said the only way was to expose it to the air: easier said than done, as the weather was cold and hardly conducive to wearing strappy tops.

Eventually the only thing to do was take to my bed every afternoon and snuggle under the bedclothes leaving my arm stuck out sideways. Slowly the wound got better, leaving a deep hole; the upside is it that it never grows hair and I don't have to use a deodorant on that side.

As you can imagine this wasn't a very happy period for us, and Jack's behaviour was getting more erratic by the day. After he had done something particularly odd I broached the subject of him seeing the doctor, and he completely lost it. He came so close to me I thought he was about to hit me. He shook with anger and started calling me all the names under the sun, using four-letter words he never used in front of men, let alone me – his wife. I had become the enemy because he couldn't pull the wool over my eyes, although he was convinced he was fooling everyone else.

From then on I walked on eggshells. I had to watch every word or it would be misinterpreted as criticism. In the past, when either of us had done something stupid we used to say "You silly old fool," almost as a term of endearment, but now that expression was taboo. If he helped me unpack the shopping I would bite my tongue as he wandered around the kitchen without the foggiest notion of where to put the bread... which was kept in a crock over a foot high with BREAD on the side. It had been in the same place for sixteen years.

Even the fridge was a mystery to him, and once when I asked him to fill the kettle he shook it at me saying, "Look, look- there's nothing in it." When I gently suggested he fill it with water he couldn't find the sink and went into the garden. He would have filled it from the water butt if I hadn't stopped him.

It reminded me of an article I'd read by Terry Pratchett, the novelist who also has Alzheimer's. Not only had he forgotten how to type, he also said that he knew his mobile was on a particular table but some days he just couldn't see it. That's exactly how Jack was at times, as if he was physically blind.

His temper became worse and worse. One day he stood in the hall swearing at me at the top of his voice, and when I reminded him of the neighbours he told me to stop swearing as if I was the one doing it. I realised he must be full of fear to behave in such a manner, but it was frightening for me too. He would have been under less strain if only he could bring himself to admit there was something wrong.

The irony of it was that for most of his life he had been very mild mannered and would never make a scene or lose his temper, even when it was warranted. This used to be irritating on occasions, but how I wished I had my old Jack back. Then he suddenly announced that he wouldn't be playing any more away games of golf. I was sorry to hear this as I knew how much he enjoyed them, but my guess was that he was having trouble finding the venues. The time had come to take matters into my own hands. If Mohammed wouldn't go to the mountain then Mohammed's wife would go instead. I made an appointment to go to the doctor on his behalf.

The doctor was kind and patient and listened without interruption as I poured out all my misgivings. Without beating about the bush he said it sounded as if Jack did indeed have Alzheimer's, but then he dropped the bombshell: he couldn't actually do anything about it unless Jack came to him of his own volition

I could hardly believe what I was hearing and my mind was in turmoil as I left the surgery. I was thankful that someone in authority had finally confirmed my suspicions, but what on earth could I do now? Jack would never agree to see him of his own accord so we had reached an impasse. This didn't make any sense to me, but was typical where mental health was concerned. If I had said that Jack had yellow fever or diphtheria the doctor would have been round to the house like a shot, so what was so different about Alzheimer's? He must have been aware that the sufferer has no sense of logic and needs to be told what to do. I suppose it must be all tied up with patients' rights or some such modem concept.

Life carried on as before with good and sometimes not so good days, and then he would do something utterly outrageous. For example, when we went to London to see my eldest son, Matthew, and his family, we stayed at a nearby hotel. (It made things easier for them and although Jack loved his little grandsons, he found them a bit overwhelming at times.) Our room was always en-suite and, like me, Jack generally had to get up in the night to go to the toilet. But he sleeps in the nude. Before you think this is too much information you will see the significance when I tell you that one night on not hearing the chain, I found him wandering along the hotel corridor completely starkers. From then on I made certain that the bedroom door was firmly locked.

One day we went to a well-known department store to get Jack some new trousers. He kept coming out of the changing room in his underpants to complain that the trousers were too short or too tight. He was completely oblivious to the other customers standing around and couldn't understand why I was making such a fuss and apologising left, right and centre. He appeared to have lost all sense of propriety.

Everything became a battle, from persuading him to get his hair cut to buying new clothes or even take a bath. I began changing his socks and pants in the night so as to avoid an argument in the morning.

He always forgot to pay the paper bills and they reached astronomical amounts before the newsagent slipped them through the letter box.

The newsagent was to figure again in an episode that caused me further heartache, and it involved the only race I ever used to bet on – the Grand National. The tradition goes back many years, when my father allowed us all to back a horse and we listened to the race on the radio. I vividly recall sitting on the kitchen stool in 1958 when my horse, Mr What, came in first, and I won the princely sum of three shillings – a fortune to me in those days.

Jack continued the custom with our own children, the difference being that we now saw it on TV, which was far more exciting. Our children might have long flown the nest but Jack and I still chose our horses, except this year, after going to place our bets, he came back saying he hadn't done so as it was so busy. I was disappointed and thought it odd, but didn't get the full story until I called in to the paper shop. The newsagent told me that Jack had come in and tried to place the bets with him. He said he took him to the door and pointed out the bookies, but Jack had turned and headed back home.

It was a silly little incident but really upsetting because it was another example of how our lives were falling apart. All the fun we used to have, the things we shared together were slipping away. I wondered how many more things were coming to an end and how much longer we could continue in this miserable fashion before one or other of us cracked up completely.

6

A Diagnosis and a Community Nurse

In November the following year, our theatre company was putting on a comedy and I offered to help with publicity. I managed to secure the use of a comer shop and put together a display of photos, some props appertaining to the plot, plus a poster with all the relevant information on it. The solicitor acting for the shop's owner warned me that it had been sold and was due for refurbishment, but the builders weren't expected to start for some weeks. So I took over the main window, with the side window being filled by the local football club with a display of jerseys, scarves and a large notice denoting future fixtures.

Two weeks later I saw that the builders were already clearing the premises and all my things had been piled in a comer with pieces of broken shelving. I was afraid they would be carted away as rubbish. I salvaged my stuff but was concerned that the football club might not be aware of the situation and some of their gear looked expensive. I wanted to take down their number on the notice and give them a ring but hadn't got a pen with me, so I asked Jack to do it while he was out on one of his frequent walks.

The shop was virtually at the bottom of our road, only three minutes away, and I gave him explicit instructions but he was back in ten minutes saying he couldn't get near the place for traffic cones. I hadn't spotted any that morning so

I asked him to try again, reiterating my instructions and even reminding him of what the shop used to sell. Again he returned empty handed.

This time I grabbed my coat and went with him and when we got there he went very quiet and had no excuse to offer. He looked sad and deflated and knew he had missed the unmissable. I seized my opportunity and said "NOW will you come with me to the doctor?" To my amazement he gave in. As soon as we got home I rang the doctor's receptionist, and then waited anxiously until the day of the appointment.

The doctor handled him with diplomacy, congratulating him on making the decision as if it had been Jack's own idea to come and making no reference to my earlier visit. He assured Jack that he had done the correct thing and to leave everything in his hands. He'd arrange for a specialist to visit us at home. The specialist would ask a few questions and then we could go on from there.

Shortly afterwards the hospital called saying the lady specialist would like to visit us the following day if that was convenient. Convenient! I had waited years for this moment. Mind you, that's not to say I didn't have mixed feelings as I put the phone down. My relief was tempered with fear that Jack wouldn't co-operate when it came to the crunch, or maybe he would come over as perfectly normal – which sometimes he was – and that she would think I was making a fuss about nothing. I hardly slept that night, although Jack slept beside me like the proverbial log.

The doorbell rang and a short, blue-stocking type of woman, hair escaping from a severe bun and glasses halfway down her nose, stood on the doorstep. She was not what I'd expected at all, but that was all to the good because Jack didn't take to high-powered women. I made a pot of tea and we sat talking about inconsequential things and suddenly she came out with it – the A word, the word I had never dared to mention. I glanced at Jack and his expression didn't change one iota, it was the same as when we had been told I had breast cancer; it was as if she was referring to a total stranger.

She asked him some basic questions: his age, how long we had lived here and what work had he done before he retired. Two of his answers were wrong and I didn't know whether to correct him or not, but remained silent. I would have liked to have had a few minutes alone with her but didn't see how this could be achieved. Then she gave him a pen and paper and asked him to draw a clock face, marking in the hours. When he'd done it, she handed it back saying did he realise that he had filled in the hours anti-clockwise? He just shrugged and gave a little laugh.

She explained they could never be 100% certain about Alzheimer's without operating on the brain, but hastily added that wasn't going to happen. Then she asked him if he still drove a car, and had he any problems with driving? Jack replied that he was fine on that score. I sat quietly and bit my tongue. She suggested that I saw a solicitor about gaining power of attorney as this was the usual thing, and then told Jack he would be contacted shortly for a memory test. She stood up, thanked me for the tea, I saw her to the door and that was it – the deed was done.

He didn't refer to the visit afterwards so neither did I, but the next day the hospital rang and asked us both to visit in three days for the memory test. A pleasant young man asked Jack thirty questions ranging from very easy to slightly more difficult ones, such as could he spell 'world' backwards. Even I had to think about that one but Jack did it straight away. He also managed to write a coherent sentence. It was the simple questions he struggled with, such as what season were we in, and what was the day and date.

The thing that shook me most was when the doctor gave him three words – ball, table and apple – saying he would ask Jack to repeat them again later. I assumed he meant at the end of the test but he asked him again almost immediately. Jack couldn't remember even when prompted. That explained everything. His short-term memory was non-existent.

The doctor told Jack he had scored twenty-five out of thirty and that he would prescribe Aricept pills. These wouldn't cure him, but they would help stop his memory deteriorating further for the time being. The doctor then went on to ask Jack how he was managing with his personal hygiene, could he dress himself and was he getting plenty of exercise. Jack ignored the first two questions but rambled on at length about how he played football and cricket and tennis and went swimming, but omitted to mention golf – which he'd played for the last twenty years. We had been married for forty-seven years and never once in that time had he played tennis. The only swimming had been with the boys when they were small.

To hear him talk you would have imagined he'd been in the last Olympics. As for baths and changing his clothes, that was all down to me. I sat there squirming with frustration, but fortunately the man handed me a questionnaire to fill in and I was able to present the true side of how matters stood.

Soon after this I was told that a community nurse was going to call on us. She seemed OK at first: there was an assessment to fill in and I was presented with a large folder full of information which mostly didn't apply to Alzheimer's. I couldn't help noticing that she mostly ignored Jack and asked me questions about him as if he was deaf, I felt very uncomfortable as I didn't want to belittle him or cause an argument.

This was the first of several visits and I began to think they were a waste of time. The nurse sat there supping tea and eating cake (she was a huge lady) and started telling me, of her own family problems, and Jack would get bored and fidgety. Once I suggested he went for a walk and she didn't object or ask him to stay. She may have been a wizard at changing dressings or physical care but I failed to see the point of these constant visits, and told her so. She replied that it gave me the chance to off load on her. I felt like saying that the boot seemed to be on the other foot as far as I could see. In the end I told her that I would contact her should I feel the need.

I told the hospital of my decision and before I knew it I was asked to come and see the head of social services. I thought I was going to be ticked off but on the contrary, he was absolutely charming. He asked after Jack and I told him how awkward I felt talking to the nurse about him as if he wasn't there. About how I didn't want to give away my secrets, such as spiriting away his clothes in the night to replace them with clean ones.

The man said I was handling Jack with great tact and apologised if one of his staff wasn't so sensitive about his feelings. He said that the community nurse in question had certain issues, intimated that I wasn't the first to complain and added that he intended to put her on a retraining course. I felt rather bad about that and said as much, but he replied that he was extremely grateful for my input. As head of department, he said he couldn't be aware of everything that went on, and he wished that everyone would speak up when they were unhappy about something.

I learnt several valuable lessons that day: that it pays to complain, and that nobody is infallible when it comes to mental illness because even the experts are still learning. So much has to come from the carer and, unlike physical illness, nothing is cut and dried and everyone is different. Even when you are given a form to fill in it is written in such a way as to cover a large spectrum of disabilities and often won't apply to the particular situation. Having said that, there's usually a space near the end for further comment. Seize the opportunity and tell it how it really is.

I was assigned another nurse who was much easier to relate to and readily agreed to come only when required, or if she had something important to tell me. She treated Jack with respect and explained things to him so that he felt included, even if he did forget everything the moment she left the house. In fact, life was getting a lot easier. Until Barrie came on the scene.

7

Barrie

Our car was getting more and more dented and scratched, and when I mentioned this to Jack he said that it was always the other fellow's fault or it had been damaged in the night, which I couldn't argue with because we parked in the road around the corner and occasionally cars did get vandalised. I was afraid Jack would have a serious accident and very much regretted that he hadn't been banned from driving at the time of his diagnosis. I think it is ridiculous to take the word of someone with Alzheimer's when asked if they are fit to drive. The community nurse even said with a laugh that they only deem it necessary to ban someone when their partner refuses to get into the car with them. All very amusing, but it needs someone in authority to make the decision and it's no laughing matter for the driver concerned – or other road users.

After breakfast one Sunday, Jack suddenly got up and said he had to go and check on the car. He came back very agitated saying that he couldn't shut the door on the passenger side. He had played golf the previous day and I think something must have happened and he had only just remembered. I suggested he should have a word with our neighbour, Jason, who went to look at it and said he didn't know how to fix it but he knew of a man who might help if we didn't want to wait until Monday and go to a garage. That was how Barrie came into our lives; a black-hearted villain with a disarming smile and a delightful Shropshire burr who was to end up costing us a great deal of money.

Jack had never been knowledgeable or interested in cars; he said they were just a means of getting from A to B. I knew even less so we were ripe for the picking, and Barrie the con-man soon cottoned on to this. He took the car away for five days before bringing it back with the door repaired.

Jack was in the habit of going out for long walks, sometimes for over two hours, but as he always found his way home and was good at crossing roads, I wasn't too worried. To be truthful I was glad of the break. Whether Barrie was monitoring us I don't know, but he always seemed to turn up when Jack was out. He'd sit in the kitchen eating biscuits and drinking coffee and blinding me with science as he explained all the things that needed doing on the car. He asked me to pay for the door, which I did, and offered to get it through its MOT. One day he lugged in the exhaust and plonked it on the floor, pointing out the state it was in and saying he would have to replace it. My common sense tells me now that exhausts probably always look filthy, but at the time he sounded so plausible I believed him

I started paying him £150 here and £200 there and it soon mounted up to a tidy sum. One of the reasons why I didn't protest was that I was anxious to get the car in tip-top condition in the hopes of selling it, so I wouldn't have to worry about Jack having an accident. He had already intimated that he was giving up driving because he wasn't going to play golf anymore. I suggested that someone could give him a lift to the course or he should speak to the captain, but he was adamant, saying he was too old. I said I knew of many older players still hobbling round the course following hip replacements, but Jack wouldn't change his mind. No doubt there was more to it than the driving, but I was never going to get the real reason.

All this time Barrie was aware of Jack's illness and that I was still having regular check-ups with my surgeon and oncologist. I've called him black-hearted, but that's not true: I don't think he had a heart at all. He even offered to run me to the hospital knowing full well I used a community car. I've wondered since what his response would have been had I called his bluff.

The penny finally dropped when he said he'd found a buyer for the car and quoted a sum of money that sounded ridiculous to me. I said I'd have to consult with my sons first before taking such a step and his whole attitude changed. He told me I was embarrassing him because he'd already made a promise to the buyer. I was in a tricky position because he still had possession of the car.

The final straw was when a neighbour told me he had seen our car in town several evenings running, and the driver was delivering the evening newspaper. When I confronted Barrie with this information he began to bluster and said he was only trying it out, that it wasn't doing the car any good for it to stand idle. I saw red and said he was taking me for a fool and that I'd never heard such nonsense and I wouldn't pay him another penny. He got really nasty and I said if the car wasn't outside our house the next day I would contact the police.

He loomed over me. I'm only five feet tall and he was at least six foot and I felt really intimidated, but I remained firm and somehow manoeuvred him out of the front door.

When I shut it I was shaking like a leaf. The next day I looked out of our bedroom window and there was our car at the kerbside, thank God!

About a week later I opened the door to a total stranger who said he was interested in buying the car. When I asked him how he knew we wanted to sell it he told me he was Barrie's mystery buyer. He hadn't been given our address but knew roughly where we lived, and had spotted the car where we had parked it overnight. He started to knock on a few doors and had eventually found us. It turned out that Barrie had asked him for £1,000 more than he told me, so you can guess who was going to pocket the difference. We came to a compromise and he bought it for a fair price and I got on to Trading Standards and reported Barrie. They weren't very interested and said that as he wasn't registered as a garage owner they couldn't do much about it, but would put him on their computer.

Jason was mortified when I told him the full story. He made a few enquiries and discovered that Barrie was actually a lorry driver who just happened to be an amateur mechanic, and that he had a bad name in the area. People are usually so kind and trustworthy in this little market town but I suppose there are always a few bad apples, and we had been unlucky enough to find one. I decided not to dwell on Barrie and put him out of my mind. In any case, I soon had something else to worry about.

8

Oh My Aching Back

During all the business with Barrie, Jack remained a bystander, content to leave everything to me, as he did with anything to do with money, changing light bulbs or dragging out the wheelie bins. The latter were particularly frustrating. I would sort all the rubbish into separate piles for our ever-increasing number of containers, only to find he had moved them back into one big heap.

Jack did occasionally make the bed (at my instigation), and he still did the washing up and prepared the bird food – but never thought to take it out to the bird table, in spite of me reminding him that they couldn't collect it from the kitchen themselves. I bought a new bird table as our current one was falling apart and stood it in the hall when it was delivered. We had some small china birds, so I placed them on the table and tied a large golden ribbon around the stand for a laugh, and waited for Jack's reaction when he returned from his walk. But he didn't give it so much as a glance. He just edged around it and went on into the front room without a word, as if it was the most natural thing in the world to find a decorated bird table in the hallway.

When he wasn't walking, Jack would sit for hours staring into space, or sometimes watch television or look at a book. His taste in television had changed; he used to be quite high-minded and would chide me for watching *EastEnders*, but now he preferred children's programmes and quizzes. If a serious play was on in the evening, he would give it five minutes before reaching for a book.

He had always been an avid reader and our house was full of books, but now he only read autobiographies, ones about wildlife or sports books with plenty of photographs. He took no interest in current affairs or newspapers, although he did keep a novel by his bedside to read at night.

He had one particular book that I had given him and I wanted to read myself afterwards, as we generally swapped books. He seemed to take forever reading it, and would often re-read a previous chapter - I assumed to keep track of the plot. After two months I couldn't stand it any longer and surreptitiously moved his bookmark nearer the end. He didn't notice, and finally finished it and passed it over to me.

For a year or so my best friend Joyce and I had been doing some entertainments for the WI and other local societies. We followed in Jack's footsteps and got on the WI speakers list and had quite a few engagements lined up. Joyce did the driving and the financial side; I was their phone contact and handled the publicity. We devised a programme of poetry and prose about Christmas, and later, one on men. We had no difficulty in finding material for the latter, the problem was to cut it down to an hour! I was loath to give this up as I didn't dare to commit to a play anymore, but felt it safe to leave Jack alone for a couple of hours in the evening because he was unlikely to venture out after dark. He even came with us occasionally, but preferred to stay at home most times.

In December 2007 we went to a WI meeting and, as was our custom, took turns to sit and stand as we performed our individual pieces. Because I knew I would shortly be standing again I tended not to sit right back in my chair, so all my weight was on my upper thighs. When I got home that night I began getting twinges in that area, but thought no more of it until the next day when I went to help at a charity shop, where I would hoover the carpets, water the pot plants and help with the window dressing.

Now the time had come round to erect the shop's artificial Christmas tree- my least favourite job. It entailed pushing all the branches into a central core, and I usually ended up with some over. The best way to tackle it was to sit on the floor and work from the bottom up. As I was doing this my back started to ache, and once I had completed the task I could hardly stand. I then had to decorate the wretched thing, which meant more bending and stretching. Finally, with the aid of a fellow volunteer, we lugged it into the shop window- all the time dropping baubles like raindrops.

Later the same week I put in several hours painting the scenery for the theatre company's Christmas show. Normally we painted standing up, but this year, for some reason, the scenery had been laid out flat on the stage, which involved further bending. By the time we had finished I felt every one of my seventy-two years. My back and legs were killing me.

I thought a few warm baths with Jack's muscle relaxant would do the trick, and although my back did feel better my legs were as bad as ever. My only means of relief was to sit or lie down but with Jack being the way he was there was fat chance of that happening as there was always plenty to do around the house. It was as much as I could manage to cook a meal Thank goodness Jack was still in washing-up mode, because I was fit for nothing afterwards other than to recline on the settee like an ailing Victorian heroine.

Shopping was a nightmare; Jack carried the bags but even with a list and a map of the shelves he couldn't find his way around a supermarket, so I would sit on a chair and issue instructions. He invariably forgot something vital and we'd end up rowing in public.

In a panic I went to see the doctor who wasn't overly helpful, saying I would have to wait three months to see a physiotherapist. He gave me painkillers to tide me over and when I protested he suggested I get some private treatment, giving me the number of a physio in my area. I hobbled to her house and in spite of my pain couldn't help smiling because there were ten steps leading up to her front door, which didn't strike me as ideal for her clients.

The physio was kind and sympathetic, but her exercises only seemed to exacerbate my condition. She tried acupuncture as well, but I wasn't improving. After several visits she admitted defeat and said that although the pains were in my thighs she thought the problem lay with my back.

I returned to my doctor and this time he suggested I see a rheumatologist – a joints specialist. He warned me it would be expensive, but I was so desperate I was ready to try anything bar amputation – my consultation lasted forty minutes. The specialist stretched and twisted my legs and I felt fine on the couch but as soon as he helped me to my feet I let out a yelp and clung to him for dear life. Like the physio he thought that my back was the real problem, and told me to get an MRI scan to get to the root of the matter. In the meantime he prescribed some little blue pills which caused me to sleep like a top at night, but I felt like a zombie during the daytime.

So it was back to the doctor again, where I begged him to book me in for a scan as soon as possible. I impressed on him that I couldn't continue in my present state, and that he would have to get Jack into a home, and me too, if things didn't improve. He promised to pull a few strings and not long after I got a hospital appointment. I was warned about the noise and the feeling of claustrophobia during the scan, and indeed it was an unpleasant experience - but there was no way I was going to push the panic button.

Instead, I lay there picturing myself in a wheelchair. The thought of having to be under Jack's control was all I needed to see it through.

The results came in the post: there was a certain amount of degenerative facet joint disease and a small cyst and a disc bulge causing narrowing of the spinal canal but there was no nerve compression or root entrapment. I was thankful for small mercies. It could have been worse, and there was no mention of the operation I had secretly feared.

I was given calcium tablets for my bones, some new painkillers, and was more or less told that either I would improve with time or I would have to learn to live with the discomfort.

Meanwhile, back at the ranch, the house was a mess and the garden was starting to resemble a jungle. I didn't know who to turn to next, until passing the door of Age Concern one day I swallowed my pride and went in to see them, pouring out all my woes in a rush.

The lady behind the desk was most considerate but said she couldn't get me a cleaner for three months and the chance of getting a gardener was even less likely – possibly in a year's time. That just about finished me and I burst into tears. The lady made me a cup of tea and said she would send a gentleman called Tom to see us. If nothing else he might get us some financial assistance, and then I could afford to pay for a cleaner to keep things ticking over until a domestic help became available. I can't praise Age Concern enough: they certainly lived up to their name. Tom came to see us within a week and quite literally changed our lives.

8

Father Christmas in Disguise

Tom was a lovely man – I used to call him Father Christmas because he arrived bearing gifts. He was dismayed to hear that we weren't getting any benefits and said that as soon as Jack was diagnosed he should have had an attendance allowance, and that I should have been getting a carer's allowance. He also looked at our finances: bank statements, Jack's company pension and our building society account – in other words all the money we possessed. He totted it up and said we were also eligible not just for a cut in our council tax but that we might not have to pay it at all.

He asked about my health. I was still hobbling and Age Concern had obviously filled him in on my aches and pains. He said I qualified for an attendance allowance as well. There was the inevitable form to fill in but he helped me with it, not missing anything out - including the fact that I had to go upstairs on all fours, which I'd only mentioned to him as an aside. Tom then suggested that I get in touch with social services, because we should be getting pension credit.

It was as if a miracle had happened. Maybe I was naive but I had no idea we were entitled to all this extra money. I had assumed that as we owned our home and had paid off the mortgage in 1983, when my father died and left me some money, we would be seen as being relatively comfortably off. Of course we were compared to some people.

Now I had power of attorney and handled all the money I was aware that our cash reserves were going down, especially with all our hospital visits and no car at our disposal. Then there were extras, such as Jack's glasses. He had objected strongly to wearing glasses so to keep the peace I had let him choose lightweight, rimless ones. These were very expensive and he promptly lost them, so I had to pay for replacements. Jack never went near a dentist, but I was constantly paying for treatment for myself as I couldn't get an NHS dentist in the town.

Jack and I both grew up in wartime and were used to seeing our parents struggle to make ends meet – they just got on with it. Then there was no hire purchase or credit cards: if you couldn't afford something you either went without or saved up for it. Time had moved on, but we hadn't. Also I must confess there was an element of pride or even snobbery in my reaction. Respectable people like us didn't ask for hand-outs. When I had gone to Age Concern I wasn't seeking money, but practical help.

I had a chat with my niece on the phone. She has a high-powered job in the NHS and she as good as told me not to be a bloody fool. She said we would not be milking the system, and pointed out that Jack had Alzheimer's and was seventy-eight, I was seventy-three, we both had diabetes and we weren't getting any younger. There was no extra money coming in and our state pensions were not going to cover all the extra expenses that would inevitably occur with Jack's illness.

She went on to say that we weren't exactly living high on the hog. We hadn't been abroad in years and our house wasn't full of expensive gadgets. I had to agree with her; my idea of high technology was an eighteen-inch television that picked up four stations, an electric typewriter and a washing machine.

She made it sound as if we lived like paupers but a lot of what she said was true. Any spare cash these days went on public transport, community cars and taxis, and it cost a small fortune to visit our sons. Our house was full of character, to use estate agent jargonese, but it was built in 1860 and there was always something that needed repairing. I used to do most of the decorating but our days of DIY were long gone, and repairs and decorations at £20 an hour were making a big hole in our savings.

My trouble is that I have a guilt complex about spending money. I used to make all the boys' clothes when they were small, and cook meals from scratch. We grew a lot of our own vegetables and I baked my own cakes - to this day I feel guilty if I buy a cake from the bakers. When Jack was made redundant I continued to be careful with money, and now I couldn't get out of the habit.

I decided I must be realistic and accept, with gratitude, all that Tom said we were entitled to. There were many ways we could make our lives easier. Jack and I had become like mother and child and I was constantly looking for ways to divert and amuse him. We started having coffee out more often, although it still seemed an extravagance when we were so near to home. We began to eat lunch out more frequently, and took the occasional trip to Cardiff or Shrewsbury. Even so it was not enough, and Jack was becoming increasingly bored.

He continued to blame me for all his shortcomings; I was bossy and just out to find fault with him. If only just once he could admit to his condition I would have been so much more sympathetic, but as it was there were times when I lost my patience with him and then felt terrible afterwards.

It didn't help when neighbours and friends met him in the street and had a chat with him and then told me, almost accusingly, that he seemed perfectly normal. What did they expect - that he should be drooling at the mouth? What they didn't know was that his conversation consisted of the weather, his national service and his cartilage operation in 1963; mention Iraq and they would be met with a blank stare. I felt like snapping back that if they met him the following day they would hear the same topics of conversation again.

He had a store of little tricks at his disposal. For example, if he saw someone from the golf club he would greet them with a jocular "Hello, young fellow," because he couldn't remember who they were.

To outsiders Jack looked physically fit and young for his age; they weren't to know that the last time he came to see me in a play he had gone home in the interval thinking it had ended. The fact that I only came on in the second half and that he hadn't seen me at all never occurred to him.

We watched a man with Alzheimer's once on TV who, although admitting to his condition, sounded perfectly lucid. When the interviewer said as much, his wife interjected and said that she was his verbal punch ball. I couldn't help myself and turned to Jack, saying that's exactly how you treat me. Why do you do it? He had the grace to look shamefaced and replied, "Because you're there." It was small consolation.

To others he appeared charming but to me he was ill-tempered, morose and defiant. I'm not belittling the strain he

60

was under. It's just that he didn't need to put on an act for me!

That's why it was such a blessing when Jenny the social worker came to see me at Tom's instigation. She asked Jack if he would like to go to a day centre once a week to give us both a break. He agreed, and it was arranged for him to go every Tuesday. What a difference it made! They had regular activities such as sing-alongs, quizzes, bingo, even painting lessons, and went out in a minibus for coffee or country walks.

The staff were wonderful and kept me informed as to what they had done that day, because Jack couldn't tell me a thing when he got home.

I paid for his dinner, tea and transport, and it was worth every penny. They picked him up at 9. 30 and brought him back after four. It meant I had a few precious hours to see friends or go to Hereford or Shrewsbury shopping or to get my hair done without having to worry about him. Jack was also eligible for week-long respites, partly subsidised by them but these didn't prove to be quite so successful.

The first time we tried it, I went to my son's house in Hove for five days. It was very hot weather and although Jack went with several changes of clothing he came back in the same pants, trousers and shirt that he went away in. I could smell him as soon as he came through the door. None of his spare clothes had been used, so I rang up to complain. They apologised and said they would look into it and ring me back.

Their explanation was that whenever they asked Jack if he needed any help, he said no. Well he would, wouldn't he? I had warned them about his personal hygiene. They said that the night staff thought the day staff had dealt with him and vice versa. As they were supposed to cater for Alzheimer's sufferers I thought this was a pretty feeble excuse.

In view of this fiasco, when he went a second time I thought things would have improved, but if anything they were worse. I rang him midweek and asked to speak to Jack Bingham, but I'm sure they put me on to someone else because his voice sounded different. Then he said he had been for a walk the evening before and I was immediately suspicious - Jack couldn't remember what he'd done five minutes previously, let alone twenty-four hours ago. When he came home, in spite of the fact his clothes were all labelled, he had three items in his bag with the name Jack but a different surname. There was also a broken bottle of shampoo that didn't belong to him that had leaked over everything.

This particular home charged £580 a week, not all paid by me admittedly, and had four stars to its name. I had a mental image of some other poor old chap protesting, "My wife said I was going home on Tuesday," which was the last thing I said on the phone to what I thought was MY Jack. If they couldn't get the basics right, what else was going on that I didn't know about? They were dealing with vulnerable people who couldn't speak up for themselves. For all I knew he hadn't even been given the correct medication The whole experience was very disconcerting and I vowed never to send him there again.

10

Money! Money! Money!

The first thing that sprang to mind when I realised how much extra money was going to come our way was to install a downstairs toilet. This may sound prosaic compared to a week in the Seychelles but believe you me, it gave me just as much pleasure. We only had the one toilet and that was in the upstairs bathroom, which was an inconvenience, if you'll pardon the pun - especially when we had guests and even more so when our small grandchildren came to stay. Jack wasn't keen on the idea as it would entail some upheaval but it turned out to be a blessing when his illness progressed.

A plumber and a builder (both neighbours) would have to create a room from scratch, so I suggested an idea that had been in my mind for some time. I asked them if it was possible to make a floor over the entrance to our cellar (we couldn't actually put a toilet in the cellar because there were eight steps leading down to it, which would have defeated the purpose somewhat). They duly came up with a solution: a trap door in the floor, so that we still had access to the cellar because although we mainly used it for storage, it did contain the electric meter. The result meant that the meter reader had to do a limbo dance to gain entry, but he took it all in good part saying he'd faced worse problems.

The workmen then took a chunk out of our dining room and put in a dividing soundproofed wall, the other walls were the original brickwork, which they plastered over. Once they'd painted the whole room it looked very smart. In fact I was so proud of the result; it was my first topic of conversation when we had visitors. "You must come and see our new toilet." Well, it was more original than; "Come and see my etchings."

Although my legs still played up when I overdid things they were steadily improving, but I had given up working for the charity shop as well as my trolley duty at the local community hospital. I contacted a firm of young ladies who blitzed the house from top to bottom, even cleaning inside windows and washing curtains. It was so satisfying to have everything ship-shape again. This tided me over until Age Concern sent me some domestic help by the name of Gill. She came for two hours once a fortnight and hoovered throughout and washed the kitchen floor, and I paid a contribution for the service.

Gill became more like a friend, and still is. She and her husband helped me install two cordless phones, one in the kitchen and more importantly one in the bedroom. A few months previously I had been struck down by a bout of vertigo which had left me stranded upstairs and physically sick. I won't go into the gory details, but the whole experience was dreadful and I vowed never to get into such a situation again. I needed an upstairs phone because even though the surgery was only over the road, Jack had forgotten how to get there. I eventually managed to request a house call, so I could get an injection and some follow-up pills.

To get back to Gill, not only was she good at cleaning but she turned out to be a whizz with technical things. She assisted me with changing correction tapes on my typewriter as my fat, arthritic fingers couldn't cope, and initiated me into the mysteries of my new washing machine. In return I was able to help her when she got into a muddle with her knitting - each to their own, I suppose. I also engaged a gardener to come twice a year to prune the bushes and cut hedges, and to pop in occasionally to mow the lawn.

As the pain in my legs got better I was able to do more and thought I should contact the authorities to inform them, as my pension credit booklet was full of dire warnings about claiming money under false pretences. A form duly arrived but I found it very difficult to fill in. They clearly weren't used to people asking for their allowance to be taken away as it was geared to people requesting one. I did the best I could under the circumstances, but when it came to listing any medical problems I'd had in the last five years it read as follows: breast cancer, a kidney problem, arthritic fingers, vertigo twice, BPPV (another form of vertigo), type two diabetes and spine deterioration.

After reading this they probably thought I should have added mental problems as well. And I hadn't even bothered to mention hepatitis B (due to a change in my cancer treatment which didn't agree with me).

Whether it was because of the form I don't know, but a young lady named Claire called on me. Her title was welfare and income officer and she metaphorically rapped me over the knuckles for attempting to rid myself of my attendance allowance. She made an assessment of our finances and phoned Swansea to cancel my request, saying: "Mrs Bingham was getting a little confused." You can say that again! Claire was to be a great help to me later on when Jack went into residential care, because the changes in benefits were a minefield and completely beyond my capabilities.

Several people suggested that now we could afford it we should go on a cruise. They meant well, but they still didn't get it. I could just picture Jack on a large liner; all the decks look similar and I wouldn't have dared to let him out of my sight. Also by now his table manners left a lot to be desired; he would blow his nose on linen table napkins and lick his spoon or knife and put it back in the communal dish of jam or butter. I could see that going down well at formal dinners. No - any money we had to play with was best spent on making our home 1ife as comfortable and rewarding as possible.

One of the reasons we were so affluent was because we received a year's back pay for Jack's attendance allowance, which he should have had when he was first diagnosed. I still can't fathom out why nobody informed us of this entitlement. Neither the community nurse, social services nor our many doctors ever raised the subject. How were we supposed to know? How many more people are missing out on benefits? It was only my going to Age Concern and Tom sorting us out that it came to light. Once you are in the system you're bombarded with information and I have a stack of booklets stating what our rights are, but heaven help those who can't speak up for themselves.

Another use for the money was to get Jack a further three days at the day centre. He was becoming increasingly restless and going out for longer and longer walks, sometimes for hours at a time. On one occasion he was out for ages. It was raining and I was on the verge of ringing the police, but I asked Joyce for her advice instead. She went out in her car to search for him, but in the meantime Jack returned. I told him that Joyce was out looking for him He said that he knew and that she had brought him back — he had come indoors and slammed the door in her face!

I eventually caught up with Joyce and apologised. She said she had found him on the outskirts of town walking up and down people's driveways.

Shortly after that incident Jack disappeared for more than three hours. This time I did call the police but he returned before they found him When I told him what I had done he just shrugged as if it was of no importance. At least he would be safe at the day centre. They could keep him occupied.

Months later I discovered by chance that sometimes he had gone into a cafe for a meal Those were the occasions I had thought he was off his food; now I knew why.

One good thing was that Jack slept well at nights, because some Alzheimer's sufferers turn night into day and that must be dreadful. Imagine if you were elderly and your partner kept you awake half the night? It must be like having a young baby all over again. At least I didn't have that to deal with.

In spite of all these little traumas I wanted us to lead as normal a life as possible. That's why in 2009 I ventured to do something that had been in my mind for some while. Our golden wedding anniversary was imminent and although my first thought had been to ignore it— there seemed precious little to celebrate — I decided to take the plunge and make some arrangements for the big day. It seemed to me it was important for Jack to meet up with all the family, possibly for the last time before his memory gave out entirely and he slipped into La-la Land.

11

Golden Wedding

Somebody told me about a lovely country house hotel near us that specialised in weddings, birthdays and anniversaries, so with Joyce in tow for moral support I made an appointment to see the manager. The hotel was run by a French family and was renowned for fine dining, and as Jack still appreciated his food I was sure he would enjoy it. Over coffee and homemade biscuits we discussed the menu and I made a provisional booking for five double rooms and a single for my brother-in-law. The manager explained that we would be eating in a small room overlooking the grounds.

I sent out invitations to all the family saying that we couldn't afford to pay for their accommodation but the meal and drinks were on us. I impressed on them not to buy any presents and stipulated no children, because, much as I loved the little ones, I wanted it to be a civilised occasion (although I didn't actually put this last bit in writing). Everyone said they could come and made their own bookings, which meant eleven of us would be sitting down to dinner. As for friends and neighbours, I had other plans for them on the Sunday.

Jack and I were shown to a luxurious room on our arrival and I changed into my best clothes and laid out a suit for Jack on the bed. I ran a bath for him and while he was soaking, popped downstairs to put out the place names, which I'd painted myself with suitable motifs. I wasn't gone more than ten minutes, but when I got back upstairs he was running along the landing without a stitch on in search of me.

I nearly had a fit and bundled him back in the bedroom before anyone saw him, but I'm positive he would have gone downstairs had I not intercepted him in time. He had the clothes he had taken off clean clothes on the bed and a fluffy white bathrobe at his disposal but he had ignored them all. He hadn't even put on a pair of underpants.

We all met up in the bar later for drinks and fancy nibbles before taking our places at the table for a memorable meal that lasted for most of the evening. Afterwards we sat in an annexe to the bar. My nephew had made a tape of songs of the 1950s, which we listened to as we had more drinks, petit fours and coffee. Some of our guests had decided to make a weekend of it but we said our goodbyes after breakfast the next day. As Miles ran us back home, I began, mentally, preparing Stage II.

I laid out a buffet in the dining room, which was laden with flowers from the family, and gathered as many seats as I could muster; fortunately the weather was kind and we were able to spill out into the garden as well. I put rugs on the lawn and the children had a picnic and played ball games and everyone seemed to have a good time, including Jack, although I'm not sure he fully understood what was going on (on our forty-ninth anniversary we had gone to a restaurant, where he kept clinking my glass and wishing me a happy birthday). Poor Jack did try and keep up with everything, and although he had stopped buying me cards and presents I would sometimes pull out a book and find a hidden card addressed to me that he had forgotten about.

This all happened in September. We followed it with a quiet Christmas, and Jack had a break from the day centre before returning in January. The next month I had a phone call to say that he was having difficulty finding the toilets and had been caught using the sinks in the laundry room They photocopied pictures of a lavatory and attached them to the toilet doors, and that did the trick for a while.

Jack began to develop what I called a prison shuffle, which although I found irritating was of no great consequence except that I was afraid he would trip up. He did fall a couple of times in the garden but didn't hurt himself; and as he wasn't going for walks so often I wasn't too worried. When he was at home he still got restless in the afternoons. Once when he went for a walk, he was back within ten minutes saying that he'd been to the market. But he couldn't have got there and back in that time.

Jack kept dropping points with every memory test, and by the end of the year he was down to seven out of thirty. I used to give him little tasks to do because he was so bored and seemed to want to be of use, but he struggled with even basic things. He couldn't make tea or coffee, and setting the table was more like rocket science to him, but he still insisted on washing up – even between courses. I don't know if I was helping by giving him jobs or being unkind, as I had no guidelines and could only trust my own instincts.

I finally persuaded him to wear boxer shorts in bed, but had to constantly remind him to put them on.

Clothes had become a mystery to him. He would cheerful wear the same thing every day, go out in the rain in a gilet, or complain of the heat when all he had to do was to remove his sweater.

Joyce and I still did our entertainments occasionally, and I'd leave Jack a prominent note saying where we were going and what time he could expect me back. He was usually in bed when I got home, even if I was early. The bedroom would feel like a sauna because he would switch on the heater the second I'd left the house.

One day Joyce and I had an engagement with a luncheon club some distance away, so we agreed to do a bit of shopping first and have our lunch out. I was being picked up at 9.45am. By then Jack should have been at the day centre, but as fate would have it they were late calling for him. They always phoned if they had a problem, so I changed into decent clothes and locked up the house, and then Jack and I were waiting in the front garden when Joyce turned up. I was in a quandary as to what to do. Jack urged me to go, and because I knew it was only a matter of minutes before the minibus arrived I took a chance and told him to wait in the garden.

Hours later, when I got home, there were three messages on the phone, from my social worker. Apparently the bus had come for Jack and they'd rung the bell and got no reply, so they set off and found him wandering down the road. When they questioned him as to my whereabouts he had no recollection of me going in the car, that he didn't know where I was and asked if I was alright. By now they had visions of me slumped on the floor, breathing my last, so they rang the day centre, who said I had never done anything like it before. So the social worker rang the police.

Oh the shame and humiliation! A policewoman had taken Jack's front door key, and she and a colleague searched the entire house (she told me afterwards that she was not allowed to do it on her own). Of course, they had found the place empty. I can't say I thought much of their powers of observation because on my kitchen calendar I had clearly written where I was going and what time Joyce was picking me up,

I appreciated their concern for me, but I felt like a terrible parent who leaves their young child to go down the pub. I was thankful that at least I had made the bed and washed up the breakfast things, but there was still a pile of cast-off clothes on the bedroom floor because I had changed in a hurry. I spent the remainder of the afternoon ringing up everybody to apologise for my transgression.

On the following Wednesday the minibus delivered Jack back home early. The driver asked for a quiet word and explained that Jack had wet himself; and they had no choice but to bring him home. I phoned the centre; they suggested I leave a change of clothing with them in case it happened again. Unfortunately it did happen again. My heart would sink if I saw him come back wearing different clothes, but he never alluded to an incident so neither did I.

I told the social worker, and she asked me if I'd like some special pants for him. I replied that I couldn't see him being able to cope with pads, but she said that the ones she had in mind looked like normal ones but had a built-in lining and could be washed and used again. The only snag was that like a baby in a nappy, he might decide not to use the toilet at all and start to relieve himself whenever he got the urge to go. I bought three pairs as a standby, but decided to wait until I felt it was really necessary before venturing to use them. Little did I realise that this was only the beginning of something that would escalate, and eventually force me to take the irrevocable step of putting him in a home.

12

From Bad to Worse

Jack's behaviour started to become stranger and stranger, and sometimes bordered on the dangerous. He had a fixation with the lock on the front door and was forever fiddling with it. He often left it on the latch, so that anyone pulling down the handle could walk straight in. Once I came downstairs to find the door ajar; only the chain across had prevented it from being open all night. More than once Jack had locked me out. I would have to ring and bang on the door for ages before he heard me and let me in.

By now his walks were getting so short it was hardly worth putting on his coat and cap. If he was at home I usually took him shopping with me – although I could get around twice as quick on my own, even with my dodgy legs. I used to get halfway down the road before realising he wasn't beside me. When I turned I would see him shuffling along some distance behind. He was still careful about crossing roads though, and would remonstrate with me if I didn't wait for the little green man.

He complained of the cold but refused to wear a scarf or gloves. I offered to buy him some fine knitted ones, explaining that they didn't have to be made of bulky leather. He used to be content to watch TV or listen to his CDs, but now he couldn't settle and kept coming into the kitchen every minute. It was getting hard for me to cook or even make a phone call in peace. He'd watch me in the garden lugging branches to the wheelie bin or sweeping the paths, but never offered to help. I think it was just a security thing: he wanted to know I was there. I didn't kid myself it was from affection – it could have been anybody.

We stayed with an old friend overnight and Jack enjoyed listening to his CDs, so I tried to get him interested again in his own collection, lovingly amassed over the years. He chose a Frank Sinatra disc. I had to put it on as he had forgotten how to work the music centre, but he lost interest almost immediately saying it went on for too long. I think if I had sat with him he would have been alright, as he was when he watched TV in the evenings, but the whole idea had been to give me a bit of space.

Jack's hearing was getting worse but when I suggested he should have a hearing test, he protested that he could hear perfectly well and that it was my fault for mumbling. If that was the case then so did most of the people on television, as he had the set turned up uncomfortably loud and I was always afraid the neighbours would complain. It was frustrating, because half the time I didn't know if he couldn't hear me or if it was more that he didn't understand what I was saying.

Finally I ignored his protests and made an appointment for him to see the audiologist at the local hospital. As I suspected, he turned out to be partially deaf in his left ear and even more so in his right. As he had previously had his ears syringed to no effect, the doctor fitted him with a small hearing aid. In the consulting room Jack conceded that he could hear better, but I had a feeling it would be a different story when we got home.

As I feared, on arriving back at the house, Jack refused to put the aid in himself; so I attempted to do it for him – only to have him complain that I was hurting him. Perhaps I was; it was difficult to gauge the correct angle, whereas if he did it himself he would know at once. I finally got the aid in as per instructions, but he kept saying it was uncomfortable and pulling it out or pretending that it had fallen out, which was impossible. I persevered for a week, but in the end I got sick of him. arguing. I said if he preferred being deaf it was up to him. He replied it was better than listening to me wittering on all the time. Happy days!

One evening I was watching a TV programme that particularly interested me, and without thinking I asked Jack to nip upstairs to pull the blinds and switch the heater on. He was gone for what seemed an age.

When I investigated, I found him in bed and refusing to come down again, although it was only 9 o'clock. I think that walking into the room must have triggered a reaction that it was bedtime. I was sure he wouldn't sleep through the night, but he slept solidly for ten hours. Time held no meaning for him: at his next memory test he couldn't identify the season, although we had walked through four inches of snow to get there. He also forgot what country we lived in. When the doctor prompted him, saying it began with an 'E', he answered Enfield - the town we had grown up in.

I knew we couldn't continue like this for much longer, but in a moment of madness or perhaps a desire to make the most of what time we had left together, I booked another holiday in the Highlands. Nearer the time I rang the hotel and asked if we could have a separate table at mealtimes, explaining our circumstances. They were very understanding, even asking if there was anything else they could do to make our stay more pleasant.

Then I had a chat with the social worker, outlining the pitfalls I could see ahead. I told her that on every trip as soon as the coach stopped, everyone made a bee-line for the toilets. The men would be out again in two minutes but as usual we ladies had to queue, and I feared that by the time I got out, Jack would have wandered off. "If only I could go with him," I groaned.

"But you can," she replied, "if you went into a disabled toilet." You see, like everyone else, I still didn't equate mental illness with disability. I thought this was a brilliant suggestion, but the social worker went on to say that disabled toilets were often locked and by the time I had got hold of a key, Jack might not have been able to wait. "What you need is a radar key," she said. "I'll get you one."

Seeing my bafflement, she explained that a radar key would unlock every disabled toilet in the country. I laughed and said it sounded like something out of Doctor Who. I imagined pointing a sonic screwdriver-like device at the cubicle and the door swinging open. I was crestfallen when the social worker said it was just a large key and only worked if the toilet was vacant so nobody could get caught on the loo.

The key really worked and I took it everywhere with me. You can get one from the council office or over the internet. With that problem solved I felt much happier about our trip, but as further back-up I decided to keep a bag with a change of clothing on the luggage rack of the coach. I also packed Jack's special pants and a good supply of trousers. I was determined to make this holiday work.

On the day before we were due to go away I went into the living room and noticed an unpleasant smell, and on tracking down the source found it was coming from our large walk-in cupboard. When I opened the door I found to my horror that everything was dripping wet and smelt of urine. I pulled out books, CDs, a set of shelves and the vacuum cleaner, all of them soaking wet. Miles, his partner Michelle and our little granddaughter were staying with us, as they were going to house-sit while we were away. They had gone for a walk with Jack, so I frantically tried to mop and sanitise before they got back. When they returned I had a quiet word with Michelle, as it was obvious from the over-powering smell of air freshener and cloths drying in the garden that something untoward had happened. I was in such a state as I still had the packing to do and this was further proof of Jack's deteriorating condition. She told me to calm down, and that she and Miles would sort it out after we had gone.

They did a marvellous job by ripping out the carpet and disposing of all the soiled things, but later in the week when Miles used the hoover it blew up, so they bought me a new one. I was so grateful for their help but at least they now knew what I had to contend with, by seeing it with their own eyes rather than hearing about my problems on the phone. In the meantime I had to get on with the packing because I had a holiday to look forward to!

13

Home Sweet Home

We managed the long journey to Fort William without incident and settled down to our usual routine. Every day the driver took us somewhere and we saw some magnificent scenery, although Ben Nevis refused to put in an appearance and remained coyly shrouded in mist for the entire holiday. Glen Nevis more than made up for our disappointment; its towering grandeur had us all craning our necks so as not to miss an inch of this spectacular ravine.

The radar key was a boon and worked its magic. I watched Jack like a hawk, as did our fellow passengers once they became aware of his illness. He nearly went to the Isle of Skye two days on the trot, but luckily a couple spotted him on the wrong coach and alerted the driver. The husband took charge of Jack while the wife intercepted me coming down the stairs with all the paraphernalia necessary for a day out.

When we got back from one of our trips we would go back to our room to change for dinner. One evening I freshened up in the en-suite bathroom and emerged to find Jack undressed and in bed. It was only 6. 15 and he hadn't washed or eaten, but I had a terrible job persuading him to get up and join me for the evening meal He was in a state of confusion for most of the time and I was permanently on red alert. I think he enjoyed the change of scenery, but on our return to Ludlow he had forgotten all about Scotland in a matter of days.

Soon it was Festival time in our market town. We attended a number of events. Jack seemed to enjoy the open-air Shakespeare at the castle and the Welsh male voice choir in the parish church, but he was bored by several of the talks by well-known personalities. These tickets had cost £17 apiece but were a waste of money, because everything went over his head and he failed to laugh at any of the amusing anecdotes they recounted. It spoilt my pleasure as we used to laugh at the same things; now we couldn't even share a joke together. The only things that amused him were TV adverts repeated ad nauseam; if I showed him a witty article in the newspaper or a funny cartoon I got no response, so in the end I gave up trying.

It must have been a month later when Jack was at the day centre and I was hoovering the living room that I noticed a wet patch on the carpet near the walk-in cupboard, and splashes on the skirting board. He couldn't get to the cupboard easily as I'd wedged a small table in front of it, hoping it would give him pause for thought. I scrubbed the patch with carpet cleaner and confronted Jack when he came home, but he denied all knowledge. Another time I caught him standing in the same area and shouted at him. He said he was removing some fluff; but it was wet again. He watched me clean up and spray as if it was nothing to do with him.

This happened about four more times. I couldn't understand why he was doing it as the downstairs toilet was only a few yards away. If he had been taken short and wetted himself in the armchair it would have made more sense to

80

me. It seemed like a deliberate action on his part. Whenever I challenged him on the subject he always said he had spilt his tea or coffee, as if I wouldn't know the difference. For me it was the last straw.

I went to the doctor by myself and told him of Jack's latest habit. He explained how Jack would have no concept of what he was doing – even if he was trying to make excuses. He asked me to bring in a urine sample to see if there was another reason for his behaviour. The result showed no physical reason why he was behaving as he was.

It was then the doctor said that perhaps it was time to think about getting him into a home. I felt sick to my stomach but in my heart I knew he was right. I was losing sleep, had no appetite and felt depressed most of the time. Our social life was now non-existent – after all, who would invite us round knowing there was a chance of Jack having an accident on their cream carpet? He even had a mishap in London when we visited our son, but luckily it was in the garden and the grandchildren were out at the time. I didn't want them to see their grandfather behaving like a child himself.

Reluctantly I phoned Jenny, my social worker, and asked her to come and see me. She was very sympathetic but agreed with the doctor and said she would post me a list of suitable homes that dealt with EMI patients- extreme mental impairment, not a phrase to cheer the heart, but I had to face up to it; that's exactly what he was. Not like the funny old local who used to say, "Hello darling. Isn't it a lovely day?" even when it was pouring with rain. With his battered hat and bandy gait he looked far madder than Jack, but he knew everything there was to know about cricket and still had a grasp on reality.

Not like the old girl down the road with her imaginary dog who still lived on her own and cooked her own meals. Jack was far worse than that and completely dependent on me. He lived in a world of his own. He was in a different league.

Jenny explained that as our total income was below £23,000 we were eligible for financial help to cover part of his fees when I found a home. This was based on an earlier assessment. When I reckoned up our present situation I was alarmed to see that due to our recent benefits we were getting about £6,000 more than that. What was I to do? Should I spend the excess and re-carpet the house? Buy some gold jewellery or pay for the holiday of a lifetime? Instead, I decided to come clean about what had happened.

Jenny put my mind at rest by explaining that the £23,000 was based on Jack's personal pension, which was very small, and half of our joint assets, this put an entirely different complexion on the situation. What a relief- but I do wish this had been fully explained to me in the first place. I might have done something very foolish and wasted money unnecessarily, and that's not to mention my sleepless nights.

I went through the long list of addresses she sent me and crossed out all the homes that were not applicable. Some were too far away for me to visit regularly; others didn't take EMI patients. Several of them had star ratings alongside their names, but Jenny said not to take notice of them as they weren't always reliable. I was forced to agree with her, because the home where Jack had gone for respite had four stars and certainly didn't merit them. The fees were variable, but it was pretty obvious that the homes in our area were more expensive than the ones in Hereford.

I started phoning the most likely prospects and it was amazing how a short phone call could give you an impression of each place. Sometimes the person who answered sounded rushed and distracted or spoke in such a strong foreign accent as to be almost unintelligible, which wouldn't do for Jack at all. Nearly all had waiting lists, and those classed as nursing homes were extremely expensive. The place nearest me asked if Jack was mobile, and when I answered yes said they couldn't take him as they weren't secure. I finally narrowed my list to five possibilities, two of them near Hereford, which I could get to by bus or train.

With the aid of my friend Joyce and public transport I made appointments to see all of them, which I did over the following weeks. The first turned out to be at the end of a long, narrow country lane, which would most probably have been cut off in winter, so that was out. Another had fifty-five beds, and the manageress locked off every corridor as she showed me around. It felt like a prison. Another smelt of toilets as soon as I got through the door, so that was out. In the end I was left with the two near Hereford, which conveniently were in the same road but were on quite a steep hill. The first one was a large, purpose-built BUPA place which was probably more than we could afford, so I carried on over the brow of the hill and arrived at a yellow-bricked Victorian villa.

As soon as I got through the door I had a good feeling about it. It was tasteful furnished but not like a hotel, the staff were friendly and welcoming and there was an air of calmness and serenity. There were only fourteen bedrooms, not all en-suite, but those without had commode chairs and there were plenty of toilets on both its floors. The huge bay windows meant the rooms were flooded with light, and there was a conservatory and a large leafy garden with no lock on the back door, so it could be accessed by the residents at any time. Margaret, the owner, was very pleasant and informative and told me that they had a range of activities on offer, their own hairdresser and pedicurist called in regularly, and there was a minibus to take the residents out occasionally. Residents could have their meals in their rooms if they desired, and the large dining room was set out with linen cloths and napkins. There were flowers and pictures on the walls. It felt like a genuine home.

I explained that I was waiting to see if I would get funding. Margaret said that they had a vacancy, but that one old gentleman was in hospital and not likely to return, so even if the vacancy was filled I shouldn't give up hope. I was so impressed that I decided I wouldn't bother to call in at the BUPA home, and asked Margaret then and there to let me know if there was a change of circumstances, and that I would keep her informed about my funding situation.

I was so pleased and excited about finding the place that my first instinct was to talk it over with Jack. But then I realised he wouldn't take it in, and if it all fell through it might do more harm than good. So I kept my silence and prayed that everything would turn out for the best.

14

If at First You Don't Succeed

It never occurred to me for one moment that my request for funding would be turned down. I had got used to the idea of Jack going away and was already planning in my head what he should take with him. When Jenny rang with the bad news I was knocked sideways, but she told me not to despair and to gather more evidence for when she presented my case again. This wouldn't be for a while as social services had only just met, so she couldn't re-submit my case too soon

She asked me if in the meantime I wanted Jack to have further respite care, but I was still so stunned I couldn't think straight so I said I'd get back to her. After thinking about it I asked her to book him in somewhere for Christmas, but not in the home he had gone to previously. Everything had to be done through Jenny, even when later I requested an extra day to allow for my travelling time. It was rather frustrating as it took up time for both me and her, but that was how the system worked.

Meanwhile, I was in limbo. I decided to see the doctor again to gather more 'evidence' for my case. My doctor was usually rather passive, but when I explained what had happened he got really worked up. He leapt out of his chair and paced the room, saying it was outrageous that I had been refused funding, that the government must wake up to the fact that there were thousands in my position all over the country and it was high time they did something about it. When I said Jack was having respite again because I hadn't used up my five-week allowance, he banged his desk and said it was ridiculous for there to be a time limit on it.

I think he was angry because it was the first time he had seen me at the end of my tether and in tears.

He even went as far as to suggest I contact my local MP, but I had another ace up my sleeve. The nurse who dealt with my diabetes was on the council and had told me if I didn't get any satisfaction, she was prepared to fight the decision all the way. Emboldened by this I rang the memory clinic and they said they would write to the doctor on my behalf. Also, without any prompting from me, my son Miles sent a letter saying he had seen with his own eyes how his Father had deteriorated and that he was concerned for my health.

I got back to Jenny and asked her to stress that I was prepared to top up his fees, because I was dismayed to find out that she had originally asked for the full amount. I had a feeling that they weren't best pleased that I had gone out of the county, although nothing was ever said in words. I couldn't see why this should be an issue as I had found a place that was £100 a week cheaper than most of the local ones – perhaps it made more paperwork for them. Another worrying factor was that she could not apply until she was certain there was a bed waiting for him.

This seemed the wrong way round to me, as with the further delay I might well lose the bed that was currently available. It made more sense to get the funding first: then at least he could be put on the waiting list. Still, what did I know about the machinations of social services?

It was now well into November and I couldn't settle to anything or even start to think about Christmas. Every time the phone rang I was expecting it to be Jenny with either good or bad news. If it was to be the latter, I hadn't a clue where to turn next. Jack was totally unaware as to what was going on and although he had agreed to go in a home, I'm sure he didn't realise all the ramifications of his decision. He thought he was going because he was old, as if everyone at eighty suddenly shut up shop and went off to be cared for.

At the beginning of December I finally got a call to say that my second request for funding had been accepted and there was still a place for him at the home of my choice. What a relief! Margaret the manageress said she would like to meet Jack before he came, and have a chat with us. I offered to take him there but she said she would prefer to meet him in his usual surroundings. She asked him a few basic questions, such as what was his work before he retired and how long had we been in Shropshire. All she got in reply was a long list of all the sports he had played. Nevertheless she said she would be happy to take him.

The date for his move was set at December the 9th, which meant everything now had to be organised in a rush. I cancelled his Christmas respite, which was a blessing because if he had gone there first and then on to permanent residential care it would have been very confusing for him. A neighbour offered to take his belongings in a van: his favourite armchair, a set of shelves for his books, playing cards and a large suitcase full of clothes. The room was furnished with the basics, but I wanted it to feel more like home. I followed close behind by car with his toiletries, family photos and his medication. I had thought of bringing along a new television, but a friend suggested that I get him one locally once he had settled in as the shop could install it. I thought this was a sensible idea.

We went up to his room, not very big, but it had a large window overlooking the garden which was a bonus. While I sorted out his clothes, one of the staff came upstairs with a tray of coffee and biscuits, which was very welcome. Then I took him down and introduced him to the other residents. By then the community car had arrived and it was time for me to go home.

As one of the carers unlocked the door Jack padded after me. I gave him a brief kiss on the cheek, not wanting to make a big deal of it. Then the thing I dreaded most happened. He tried to follow me out, completely forgetting that we had just unpacked all his things upstairs. I explained that he was staying behind. Another carer led him away and into the lounge, but I was pretty choked up as I got into the waiting car. Fortunately the driver read my mood and didn't try to engage me in bright conversation, as I was fighting back tears all the way home.

My life had revolved around Jack for so long that although I had wanted this to happen, part of me felt empty and lonely. I didn't think I would be able to sleep, but I must have been mentally exhausted because before I knew it the light was streaming in through the window and it was morning. I made my breakfast and took it upstairs with the paper, realising that I didn't have to get up early for any reason. No-one was picking Jack up; I didn't have to sort out his clothes or see that he brushed his teeth. It was very strange, almost as if he had died, but it had its compensations. Now it was up to me to readjust, to seize the opportunity to restart my life.

15

Change of Circumstance

If I thought that life was going to be more peaceful once Jack was settled, I was in for a big shock. For a start I had great difficulty sleeping at nights. Winter had settled in early, my Christmas plans were destroyed and I kept waking up feeling cold. For fifty-one years I had slept beside a warm body; now, in the worst winter for years, I was alone in a double bed. Finally I solved the problem by pulling down Jack's pillow and tucking it in the curve of my spine. This proved so successful that I kept forgetting he wasn't there anymore. Several times I tip-toed to the bathroom so as not to disturb him.

I also had to come to terms with cooking for one. My appetite was never that good, but Jack's appreciation for a good meal made all the effort of cooking worthwhile. Now I found myself snacking and convincing myself that beans on toast was an adequate dinner. Shopping for one wasn't easy either, and I had so many leftovers the garden birds were in danger of becoming obese. I put myself off sardines for life by piling them so high on toast so as not to waste any that I haven't touched them since. A tin of tuna would last me three days, so I got sick of that as well. Now I've got into the habit of cooking for two, sticking half in the freez.er and trying not to forget about it.

All my benefits disappeared like dew before the sun, including Jack's attendance allowance and my carer's allowance. My pension credit was slashed in half. All of Jack's state pension apart from £22.60 went to social services for his fees, and I was contributing nearly £300 a month as well. This added up to a considerable amount and hardly fitted the description of "topping up". Fortunately I had a cushion of money from our previous largesse, but it was difficult to tell if I was managing well or not. I had been told that should I get into difficulties they would re-assess me, but I imagine that would only be after I had used up our money in the building society.

On the plus side, Jack had settled in well and I was more than happy with the care he was receiving. In view of all the horror stories doing the rounds I was sure I had made the right choice of homes. As far as I was concerned there was only one snag: it took me nearly an hour both ways when I visited him every week (by car it only took half an hour, but the little bus I travelled on called at all the outlying villages, and I still had a fifteen minute walk up a hill). Having said that I was grateful for my free bus pass, and the driver was willing to drop me off between stops to save me a few extra yards. I also took a great deal of pleasure from the beautiful scenery on the way.

I normally arrived at the home at about 11.15 in the morning. They had lunch at 12.30, so I would be given a free meal, much appreciated, and it gave me a chance to do something normal with Jack. Before that, weather permitting, I would get him out in the garden. We would walk around while I pointed out the various trees and plants. It was amusing at first because he used to complain about it being neglected; he got it into his head that "they" had made a start and then taken the money and done a runner, as he put it. I tried to explain that "they" were actually Margaret and her husband, and that they couldn't do much because of the time of year. Our own garden looked pretty much the same. Nobody could do anything until spring.

In fact our conversations must have sounded like a sketch from the Two Ronnies. We took it in turns to speak, but as fast as I said one thing he would go on about something else, and then when I changed the topic to his he would go off on another tangent. The summons to dinner would come as a welcome relief; but even that had its bizarre moments.

Rounding up the residents for a meal took some ingenuity. Like small children, they only had to be told it was dinner time for them all to want to go to the toilet. This involved sorting out whose need was the most urgent. Eventually a slow queue shuffled into the dining room and they were all seated at tables, handbags looped on backs of chairs and Zimmer frames stacked to one side. The staff went to great pains to get everyone together for a meal It once took three of them to get one old lady to her seat because she couldn't use a Zimmer, but they were patience itself and cut up her food and gave her a spoon to eat with.

There were linen tablecloths and napkins and on St David's Day they were changed to yellow and green, and there were paper dragons on the tables. Likewise everything was red, white and blue on the week of the royal wedding. I couldn't help but wonder how many of the residents appreciated the fact – Jack hadn't got a clue as to who was getting married although I had told him several times. I was in awe of all the trouble they went to.

Sometimes several of the residents turned up their noses at the food on offer, although the staff were careful to remember who didn't like peas and so on. It made me exasperated that, like small children, they wouldn't even try a mouthful. I noticed when they took orders for tea there was usually a choice of soup or sandwiches. I thought it odd, but I suppose it was a cunning way of getting something nutritious down them. The room was always warm and the ones that complained the most about being cold were the ones that ate the least. I doubt if I would have had the patience to deal with them day after day.

Dinner was often punctuated by someone bursting into song or reciting a poem or complaining that they hadn't had a drink or had lost their napkin, which was invariably on the floor. Little quarrels broke out occasionally for no good reason, but as usual the staff handled them with tact and good humour.

After a while I got to know all the residents and became used to their funny little ways. Most of them started to remember me, but a few would always inquire as to who I was and I had to re-introduce myself as Jack's wife. At least he still remembered me, thank God, although he always seemed amazed to see me.

Violet was very friendly and was always telling me that she wanted to go home – but the home she meant was the home of her childhood with her mother and father, who were sadly long gone. Marion told me she was very athletic as a child and recounted doing exercises one day on the beach when a gentleman asked her father if she was filleted.

I thought this was amusing, but she then repeated the story using the same words, voices and inflections ad nauseam until I excused myself and went to talk to someone else.

Min, for some reason known only to herself; took a violent dislike to Jack and was always making disparaging remarks about him. The staff thought that she didn't like men with beards. I got so fed up of this that I decided to have a tactful word, being careful not to upset her. One day, after she was being particularly obnoxious to everyone, Liz, the carer on dinner duty, grabbed her pudding and said she must eat it in the lounge. Like being sent to the naughty step, I suppose. As she propelled herself through the door I heard Liz say that if she couldn't behave she wouldn't get her nice birthday tea on Friday. When I asked how old she was going to be I was told ninety-nine; I had second thoughts about speaking to her after that!

Another person that Min had taken against was Sarah. I found Sarah very interesting; she was only two years older than me, nippy on her feet and usually quite with it. That was until the day when she took me to one side and told me that her brother and his associates would be able to "clear up this mess". I had no idea what mess she was referring to, but she went on to say that his firm had branches all over the country. I expected her to hand me a business card at any moment. I think she must have been on a lot of committees in her day and sometimes had imaginary meetings with her son, the local MP and the Bishop of Hereford on the days I was there.

Sarah had her uses as she often took a turn around the garden, and Jack would go with her. He wouldn't go in the garden on his own, or even into the conservatory unless there was someone in sight. I could understand him not wanting to be in the TV lounge all the time, but he spent a lot of the time just sitting in the dining room, staring into space. He joined in the set activities every day, but the staff couldn't persuade him to read or move about. So they left him with the radio playing softly, just having the odd word with him now and again. He seemed perfectly happy and I have to be honest, the last few years he was home with me he seemed to prefer his own company.

One curious incident was when someone reported him passing over money to Sarah. He only had loose change in his pocket and when the staff checked his wallet it was empty, so he must have handed her notes. It was an awkward situation as they could hardly frisk her, but from then on they took charge of his wallet. I topped it up when necessary for haircuts and chiropody. Some weeks later I was chatting to Sarah and she told me that she sometimes did a collection for Cambodia. I informed the staff and they were pleased to have an explanation for what had happened, although where the money actually went we shall never know.

If all this sounds as if I spoke more to the other residents than my own husband, it's because he didn't speak to me very much. He often wandered off and left me high and dry. I think he forgot I was there half the time. He still recognised me when I arrived, but I wasn't part of his world any more. He showed no interest in what I had been doing all week, although I tried to keep him up to date with what had been going on. He was still eating and sleeping well, and apart from the occasional strop about washing and cleaning his teeth was behaving well.

In the meantime I was still trying to adapt to my new life, but I had no idea that my change of circumstance was going to stir up such a financial hornet's nest. I used to enjoy the sound of letters landing on my doormat; these days I dread picking up a brown envelope with Department for Work and Pensions on the top as it is usually the harbinger of trouble!

16

It never rains but it pours

At the beginning of the year I had a raft of expenses to deal with, starting with the replacement of the living room carpet that Jack had urinated on. Then of course I had to get new curtains as they no longer matched, and were eighteen years old and looked it. Then the top of one of my fillings fell out and the dentist flatly refused to patch it up again, so that meant a new one at a cost of £120.

Just to be perverse, my old gas cooker finally gave up the ghost and a new one cost me £250. I wasn't at all happy with the grill so I succumbed to a toaster, and that together with the cost of installing the cooker bumped the bill up by a further £80. Then the first of my little surprises from the DWP arrived saying they had overpaid my pension credit and I now owed them £487.

To further complicate matters I decided to change my bank to one on the high street. My previous bank had been taken over by one with a poor reputation and trying to get through to them on the phone was a nightmare, so it made sense at the time. A charming lady talked me through the procedure but it took two hours. Then she said I'd be sent a load of information through the post that I wouldn't understand, and I was to bring it in to her and she would explain it. She'd obviously got my measure but this took another hour, and I was rapidly losing the will to live. I wanted to get Jack's account – that was already with the bank – transferred to mine, but she said that was a whole new ball game involving my power of attorney and so on. I felt I just couldn't face it for the present. It is something I need to do in the future because that way I can see at a glance how much money we have between us.

I had informed the DWP of my change of circumstances as soon as Jack went away, as I was fully aware from the dire warnings issued that I would be in deep trouble should I fail to do so. Claire, my financial guru, assisted me with this, and I thought we had covered everything. My first invoice from the home amounted to more than £2,000 for several months' care. The next payment would be for one month at £286.24, reverting to a round £286 afterwards. I'd rung my bank to set this up as a standing order, asking them to knock off 24p after the first payment. They said they couldn't possibly do anything as straightforward as that and that I would have to contact them again for the second and subsequent payments, which I duly did, reminding them the first amount was a one-off.

I assumed that was all done and dusted, but after three months with my new bank I realised from my statements that I was still paying both amounts. In a panic I called in at the bank. I wanted to discuss the matter with Margaret first but she was on holiday in Ireland, so on Claire's advice I cancelled the first amount.

In the meantime, every time I got a bank statement the money out column was chock-a-block and there was nothing coming in except Jack's pension from his old firm. There was no state pension, no pension credit or my attendance allowance. I realised that at that rate I would soon be in the red. I rang the DWP and was casually informed that my notification of my change of circumstance had gone to the wrong department, but that I would eventually receive the whole amount owing on June 20th. This added up to in excess of £1,000. I was furious that they hadn't informed me of this earlier. Thankfully I wasn't having to cover a huge mortgage.

I'm pleased to say that the money did come through on that date, while Margaret returned from holiday and checked her accounts online, reimbursing me with many apologies. What else can go wrong, I wondered? I didn't have long to wait; two weeks later a thud on the doormat turned out to be nine brown envelopes all headed 'DWP'. I tore them open and couldn't believe my eyes; they all contained an identical letter saying my new pension credit would be paid into my account shortly, and I was to expect a separate letter explaining how it had been worked out. I thought I must be going insane.

Seven days later I received two more of these identical letters despite the fact that I had rung them to explain what was going on. All they said was that the computer must have had an off day. When I asked as to why nobody had spotted the error, they said airily that everything was mechanised these days. So much for progress – what a waste of time and money. It hardly filled me with confidence and when I finally get news of my pension credit, how can I be sure that they've got it right?

But to get back to Jack. Margaret informed me that none of his medical records had been passed over to her. If he should suddenly be taken ill they had nothing to refer to. He was still having his medication for type two diabetes because I had given her his pills when he went in. They had renewed his prescriptions, but he was well overdue various tests for blood and urine, not to mention special eye and feet examinations.

Even more concerning was that he still hadn't had a memory test and was still on Aricept, which I was told he should come off under controlled circumstances. The pills were of no further use to him and might be doing him more harm than good. As Jack had now been in care for more than six months and they cost £2.50 a tablet, I'll leave you to do the maths. What a waste of money when we are always being reminded that the health service is short of cash.

Margaret had made several attempts to locate his records and had come up against a brick wall, so I marched to my surgery and demanded to know why they were holding them up. They told me that his records had gone to Hereford health authority on January 20th, with confirmation following that they had arrived. It was back to Margaret who phoned them again – and they admitted they had them so they had been sitting on them for six months! Frightening isn't it? They were fifteen miles away but somehow Jack had slipped through the net. Since then he has received an appointment for his eye test but still no sign of a memory test, and they must continue to give him his pills until told otherwise. His feet have still not been examined.

This week I received a letter stating that the £22.60 that Jack is allowed after the rest of his state pension goes towards his fees has been in suspension since April because they didn't know where to send it. I suspected as much, but because all the money that goes into my account is in bulk it was hard to tell. I've made yet another phone call to give them my bank account details and hopefully I will get a rebate shortly.

I'm the first to admit that I'm not very good where financial matters are concerned but I never dreamt I would have so many problems, most of them not of my making. As Claire said, "It could only happen to you." I can't help but wonder how many other people are in a muddle, and worse still, how many more don't realise things are going wrong? My advice is to check everything continuously, never throw anything away and don't assume that the powers that be know what they are doing. Because I'm living proof that they don't.

17

To Sum Up

So what have I learnt over these last eighteen years? Have I any pearls of wisdom to impart? Only that you must learn to bury your pride and take whatever help you can get, but it's best to ignore advice from friends who haven't experienced Alzheimer's at first hand.

I can't stress enough, never throw anything away: hang on to diaries, calendars or whatever you write your day-to-day jottings on. I've lost count of the number of times I have had to refer back for doctors, the DWP and social workers.

Age Concern, or Age UK, as it is now known, is a fount of practical help and should be your first port of call for general advice and financial problems.

Day centres are a godsend and will give you and your loved one a much-needed break. They are run by dedicated people, so take full advantage of them.

Above all don't be a martyr; you can only do so much before seeking professional help. I've seen numerous programmes or read articles where family members have vowed to go on caring for someone come what may, but remember you are not dealing with a physical illness, you will receive no thanks or appreciation, in fact may only get hostility in return. You still have your own life to lead and perhaps other responsibilities. There is little point in letting this terrible illness ruin everyone's lives.

It sounds awful but you must face the fact that your loved one has become a stranger and, rather like an animal, requires only warmth, good food and a safe environment to reside in. It doesn't have to be YOU who supplies these creature comforts. When you feel that you can't go on any longer there is no shame in finding a good home for them

People say I shouldn't feel guilty and in all honesty I don't, as I know I have done my best for Jack. I am no saint. I firmly believe he is in the best place for him at this stage of his life.

I visit him as often as I can, usually once a week. He still knows me but has no concept or interest in my life away from him. I must come across as that bossy little woman who turns up from time to time and insists that he gets his hair cut or walks round the garden. I'm not even sure that he likes me anymore.

Sadly, although his sons and families visit him when they can, he doesn't appear to know them. When we introduced him to his latest grandson, born last June, it could have been any baby off the street.

When your friends invite you for a coffee don't burden them with your woes, or they will cease to invite you. Save them for your community nurse or social worker; it is all part of their job and they can shrug it off at the end of the day as they are nor personally involved.

I haven't mentioned carers' societies, where you can meet people in similar circumstances. I must admit they hold no interest for me. Just as when I had cancer, I prefer to mix with people as far removed from my problems as possible – but that's not to say they can't be of use if you have no family members to talk to.

Don't beat yourself up if you say unkind things in the heat of the moment. We are all human and can't help blowing up at times. While you are castigating yourself; the recipient of your outburst will have forgotten it in moments, so don't give yourself a hard time.

It is vitally important to keep on top of the financial side of everything. Don't assume that those in authority are always in the know; it is often the case that the left hand doesn't know what the right hand is doing.

Changing to more mundane matters, when you find a good home don't rush into things. Your natural instinct will be to make everything as familiar as possible but it is best to wait a while. I am thankful that I didn't buy a new TV for Jack as he doesn't spend any time in his room, other than to sleep. All the books I provided have remained unread, and the bedside clock I bought was unnecessary as he never consults it and is always called for his meals.

I used to take him fruit or sweets but I generally ended up throwing them away on my next visit, so now I take him a single pear or apple and see that he eats it while I am with him. I do take the occasional box of biscuits or some flowers, but that is for the home in general as a small thank you for my free dinners. I still feel lonely at times, especially when I see a programme on TV that I know Jack would have loved. I have to force myself to eat regularly and healthily as it is all too easy to exist on snacks when you have no-one else to cook for. I remind myself that there are plenty of people in the same boat as me and that I must look to the future, even if it will be different to the one I had always imagined.

18

P.S

It is now getting on for three years since Jack went into a residential home in Herefordshire. An awful lot has happened since that time so it seems only fitting to update you as to how matters stand today in October 2013.

After Jack settled down I decided to pick up my theatrical interests but it was not to be. My theatre company, that had been going for over forty years abruptly folded. I knew they were struggling and unable to form a committee due to illness and sheer old age but my hands were still tied so I was unable to be of help.

Even so, it still came as a shock. I felt as though I had lost a limb having belonged to a company since the age of fifteen.

My one consolation was that I finally was in a position to accommodate a Shakespearian actor from the Ludlow Festival.

The organisers asked for volunteers every year but with Jack being the way he was it was impossible for me to oblige.

In 2011 they put on Twelfth Night starring John Challis as Malvolio and I had a charming Irish man to stay who was always ready to have a bit of craic or intelligent conversation as I called it. Mind you his Northern Irish accent was so strong I had difficulty in understanding him at times. In the play he took two roles, one in his own accent and the other in broad York shire. When he asked me if the latter sounded convincing I replied that it did; so much so that the audience probably thought his Irish was assumed.

Last year I had the leading lady from *Much Ado About Nothing* for three weeks. She was a lovely talented girl and we got on like a house on fire. The weather was appalling and her wellington boots remained in my hallway for the entire time.

They only cancelled one performance and that was when their dressing room quarters were under ten inches of water. Ah! The joys of open-air theatre.

Unfortunately, what with the recession and two years of bad weather, the Festival lost thousands of pounds and they finally announced they were closing after over fifty years.

This was terrible news, not only for me but the entire town as it brought in a lot of business from all over the world. They are now trying to cobble together a short programme for next year just to see how things go but in the meantime we've lost Shakespeare at the Castle which was the jewel in the crown. Talk about when one door closes another shuts in your face.

Whilst all this was going on I longed to discuss it with Jack who at one time would have been as devastated as I was. He was turning into a recluse, refusing to join in the daytime activities and spending a lot of time in bed and then coming down four times a night. He had reached the phase I had been dreading when he was at home with me. When I asked the staff why they didn't sedate him at night they said they were afraid he would wake up in a befuddled state and have a fall.

Several other residents were deteriorating too. Poor Violet who wanted to be home with her parents died and

Sara, who used to be lively and on the ball, was far more subdued, but Min reached her hundredth birthday and was just as unpleasant as ever. Jack finally had all his diabetic tests apart from his eyes. We discussed it and decided he would never keep still long enough to be examined properly. Far worse was that I had to face the fact that he really didn't know me anymore. I was still vaguely familiar to him but he didn't know me as his wife and whereas I used to be able to persuade him ·to have his hair cut etc. I didn't hold any sway over him now.

The staff told me that it was increasingly difficult to shower and dress him and although he used to be happy in his own little world he was now more agitated and had what they referred to as his black days. At times he didn't use his commode or a toilet appropriately and seemed totally oblivious to the unpleasant smell in his room.

By October his behaviour became even more erratic; he threw his bedding onto the landing every day and once I got an S.O.S to bring in more shoes. He had thrown his others onto a flat roof and they could only recover one of them. He also ate the entire top off a bar of soap!

He started hallucinating and someone called Charlie appeared on the scene. He talked to him constantly and if I helped him down the stairs or zipped up his jacket he would say ' Thank you Charlie' to me. The staff asked me if he had ever known anyone by that name but although I wracked my brains I couldn't recall him mentioning him before. He could have met him at Infants school for all I knew.

The doctor examined him and managed to get a urine sample but he frightened the life out of the district nurse when she tried to get blood from him. He shouted at her and tried to grab the needle and she had to give up. The doctor said he would make an urgent appointment with the specialist but as Margaret remarked caustically 'What does urgent mean these days.'

How right she was. First we were told that the specialist was ill and then he took a holiday before returning to a backlog of work so he never saw Jack at all. Shortly afterwards, Margaret took me on one side and said they couldn't cope with him any longer. She felt they were unable to meet his needs and it wasn't really fair on her staff. In order to bring matters to a head she formally gave Jack four weeks' notice. I knew that she wouldn't turn Jack out into the snow but something had to be done and she'd given up pleading with social services.

Hilary (Jack's social worker) rang at least twenty nursing homes and I visited several but couldn't find anything suitable. One was at Clee Hill, a high remote area inhabited mostly by sheep and I nearly died of cold waiting for the two hourly bus. They had a very small landing but said he only had to ring a bell for someone to escort him down in the lift but I knew Jack would never remember to do that and I could picture him walking back and forth like a caged animal.

Another had a foyer like a grand hotel, complete with fountain and an entire wall devoted to an aquarium which he wouldn't have appreciated and the fees were horrendous. What he really needed was a mental home or a hospital ward but they were all closed in favour of 'Care in the Community', a cosy expression that meant passing the buck or saving money as far as I could make out.

Just before Christmas I was summoned to a meeting at his home. Those present were Margaret, myself, a lady who dealt with long term care and Hilary, who I had never met in the flesh before and had only spoken to on the phone. We waded through forty seven pages ticking boxes where appropriate with regard to his mobility, comprehension, general behaviour, etc. I couldn't help thinking twenty minutes conversation would have covered all of it but it had to be done by the book. Also his condition was deteriorating all the time and in a matter of weeks our findings would be out of date.

Hilary announced that she had found a possible home in Shrewsbury and that he may be moved over the Christmas period. I had arranged to be with my son in Brighton for the holiday but Margaret assured me that they would handle the move and she could ring me if it transpired.

As I didn't hear anything it was no surprise to be told that nothing had happened when I returned. Hilary told me that Shrewsbury had decided not to take him after all. As she said, given a choice, they would prefer a little old lady who sat in her chair singing to herself all day than a large man with dubious personal habits who wandered around shouting and refusing medical help. They were in a position to cherry pick

On January the 24th, 2013, social services informed me that Jack was being transferred to a nursing home in Shropshire the next day. It was in a village outside Bridgnorth and one we had discounted originally as it was too difficult for me to get to but the situation was desperate. Margaret was now at her wits end and Jack had done something so obnoxious I won't even put it into print and even I didn't get the full story until weeks later,

By then I wasn't very well myself with the remains of a cold and conjunctivitis. so I wasn't involved with the move but the nursing home rang me to say he had arrived safely .

I offered to visit as soon as I could arrange transport but they suggested I leave it a few days until Jack had settled. Ten days later, Paddy, the friend who helped me when I had cancer, took me there by car and it took us over an hour. The home was sited over seven acres of ground but all the E.M.I patients were together on an upper floor overseen by several men and a retinue of young, female staff, mostly foreign.

They were all very pleasant and helpful and Jack's bedroom was spacious with an en-suite bathroom and a view of fields and a fast running brook. I was invited to have dinner with them but I'd arranged to treat Paddy for lunch, the least I could do to cover her petrol money. Many of the patients had physical illnesses as well as dementia and had to be hand fed. I have to admit I found it depressing and rather overwhelming. I tried to talk to Jack about the horses we could see in their winter coats but got no response.

Afterwards I had a chat with the head man in his office. He told me that Jack was urinating all over the place and was having two-hourly toilet training. (This didn't work out and he is now padded up all the time.) He asked me about Charlie and was he a dog and I heard myself saying that he was a person and then explained that I had no idea who he was except that he was human.

I've managed several visits since with the aid of a circle of friends but I dread going there. I don't know what to do with myself, time passes slowly and I can't escape to the small enclosed garden .

The second in charge rings me from time to time and usually it isn't good news. Jack keeps getting urinary infections and has had several falls. This is because he keeps pacing the corridors all day. They do their best but can't strap him down or follow him continuously. They have now changed his room because he keeps fiddling with the coded lock. If by chance he should hit the correct number he could escape and would probably fall down the stairs.

With regard to the fees, Shropshire Council is footing the bill apart from taking most of his state pension which is a great relief. At £650 a week my savings wouldn't last very long.

They asked me to make up a memory board for him so I did two. One was all family photos and our wedding pictures and the other consisted of us acting in plays and an example of his writing plus one of Bayswater Road where Jack helped me sell my pictures every Sunday for many years. He used to love being in London and mixing with all the artists. This created quite a buzz with the staff and helped to show that once he was a real person with a life.

Now it is October and from always being on the move Jack is now confined to a wheelchair. There is nothing wrong with his legs or feet but his brain can't tell him how to put one foot in front of another. The staff tried him with a walking frame previously but he didn't understand what was required and continued walking holding it aloft and clinging to the wall rail with his other hand.

Now he has a chest infection and has practically stopped eating. He has a nasty graze on his forehead and has been given a bed with rails. I have had to sign numerous forms about all this and they even have a photo of his graze; I suppose they are in fear of litigation. I'm afraid it looks like the beginning of the end, looking at his memory boards I feel very sad. I still find it hard to come to terms with the fact that this talented, intelligent man is now a shambling wreck. It is a cruel disease.

I'm convinced a cure will be found for Alzheimer's eventually but it will be too late for Jack. I have willed his brain to Alzheimer's Research and mine too as they need normal brains as a comparison and I've nothing else worth taking at my age.

According to the statistics, there are 50,000 sufferers in care homes at this moment as well as those still in their own homes and that doesn't include those that are still undiagnosed. We hear so much about cancer and heart disease but mental health is still the poor relation. I'm sorry to end on such a downbeat note but Jack's story was never going to have a happy ending. My only wish for him now is that he will slip away quietly and suffer no pain. His sons are going to visit him shortly. If reading this account will be of help to people in a similar circumstance then at least some good has come out of a sad situation and I haven't wasted my time over the last three years.

*

Jack died peacefully on the 9th May 2014 at Bradeney House.
His brain went to Alzheimer's Research before cremation at Hereford,
on May 30th. He was eighty-four years old.